Candida albicans - Epidemiology and Treatment

Edited by Payam Behzadi

Published in London, United Kingdom

Candida albicans - Epidemiology and Treatment
http://dx.doi.org/10.5772/intechopen.1001505
Edited by Payam Behzadi

Contributors
Anthony Guillermo Merino Estrella, Azar Bazrgaran, Brigitte Carolina Guerra Espinoza, Charalampos Proestos, Esperanza Duarte-Escalante, Fabiola Avelino-Flores, Farahnaz Hatami, Hamed Aramjoo, Javier Aquiles Hidalgo Acosta, Jorge Eduardo Bejarano Macias, Karen del Carmen Morales-Ramírez, Mariuxi Vanessa Viteri Herrera, María Fernanda Calderón León, Nataly del Carmen Quisiguiña Jarrin, Paola Vanessa Solorzano Acosta, Payam Behzadi, Pia Afzelius, Pouria Mohammadparast-Tabas, Raúl Avila-Sosa, Ricardo Munguía-Pérez, Seyedeh Masoumeh Ghoreishi, Silvio Paul Carlosama Ruiz, Simasadat Seyedjavadi, Sobhan Mortazavi-Derazkola, Teresa Soledad Cid-Pérez, Wendy Belén Iguasnia Guala, Zahra Jahanshiri

First published in London, United Kingdom, 2024 by IntechOpen
IntechOpen is the global imprint of INTECHOPEN LIMITED, registered in England and Wales, registration number: 11086078, 167-169 Great Portland Street, London, W1W 5PF, United Kingdom

British Library Cataloguing-in-Publication Data
A catalogue record for this book is available from the British Library

Additional hard and PDF copies can be obtained from orders@intechopen.com

Candida albicans - Epidemiology and Treatment
Edited by Payam Behzadi
p. cm.
Print ISBN 978-0-85466-248-7
Online ISBN 978-0-85466-247-0
eBook (PDF) ISBN 978-0-85466-249-4

For EU product safety concerns:
IN TECH d.o.o., Prolaz Marije Krucifikse Kozulić 3, 51000 Rijeka, Croatia,
info@intechopen.com or visit our website at intechopen.com.

Meet the editor

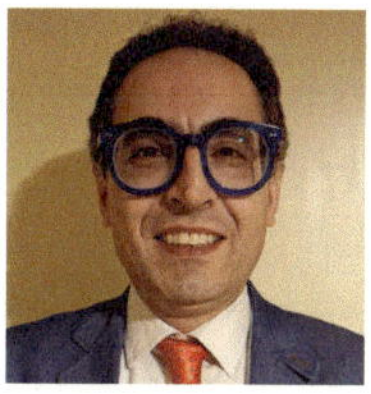

Assistant Professor Dr. Payam Behzadi has been a faculty member of the Department of Microbiology, College of Basic Sciences, Shahr-e-Qods Branch, Islamic Azad University, Iran, since 2004. He was named a Distinguished Researcher there in 2023. He has a BSc and MSc in Microbiology and a Ph.D. in Molecular Biology. He was listed among the world's top 2% of scientists in 2023 by Stanford University, USA. Recently, Dr. Behzadi collaborated as a co-author on the Global Burden of Disease Study.

Contents

Preface

Candida albicans, as part of the microbiome, plays a role in maintaining the homeostatic condition of the human body. However, *C. albicans* can become an opportunistic pathogen when homeostasis is disrupted. Both *C. albicans* and non-*Candida albicans Candida* (NCAC) possess a variety of virulence and antifungal resistance genes, enabling them to cause fungal infectious diseases [1, 2]. These clinical and pathological characteristics make *C. albicans* and NCAC significant fungal opportunists in infectious diseases.

This book presents a comprehensive overview of *C. albicans*. It is organized into three sections. Section 1 includes Chapter 1, "Introductory Chapter: Candidiasis and Antifungal Drug Resistance Feature".

Section 2, "Pathogenesis and Treatment", includes three chapters: Chapter 2, "*Candida albicans*: Pathogenesis and Secretory Pathways"; Chapter 3, "Invasive Candidiasis Due to *Candida albicans* and Its Treatment"; and Chapter 4, "Environmental and Social Determinants Related to Candidiasis".

Section 3, "Antifungal Drugs and Nanomaterials", includes Chapter 5, "Antifungal Resistance in *Candida albicans*" and Chapter 6, "Nanomaterial against *Candida albicans*".

I would like to thank the contributing authors for their excellent contributions. I am also grateful to the staff at IntechOpen for their exceptional support and cooperation, especially Publishing Process Manager Ms. Antonija Grgeč. Additionally, I extend special thanks to my fantastic colleagues Dr. Pia Afzelius and Prof. Charalampos Proestos for their brilliant collaboration on Chapter 2, "*Candida albicans*: Pathogenesis and Secretory Pathways".

Payam Behzadi
Assistant Professor,
Department of Microbiology,
Shahr-e-Qods Branch,
Islamic Azad University,
Tehran, Iran

References

[1] Afzelius P, Proestos C, Behzadi P. *Candida albicans*: Pathogenesis and secretory pathways. 2024

[2] Behzadi P, Behzadi E. Modern Medical Mycology and Opportunistic Pathogenic Yeasts. Tehran: Persian Science & Research Publisher; 2011

Section 1

Introduction

Chapter 1

Introductory Chapter: Candidiasis and Antifungal Drug Resistance Feature

Payam Behzadi

1. Introduction

Although *Candida* species, including *Candida albicans* and Non-Albicans Candida (NAC), form a portion of the human body's normal flora and act as commensal microorganisms, they can be activated as opportunistic pathogens in individuals with weak immune systems, e.g., old people, immunosuppressed individuals, and in in-patients. The natural habitats of these candidal microorganisms in human host bodies are the oral cavity, gastrointestinal tract, genital tract, and the skin, for the most [1–5]. The imbalanced overgrowth of *Candida* yeasts or their penetration into the deep tissues and organs in human host body may lead to the occurrence of life-threatening candidal infections in the bloodstream, heart, brain, kidneys, etc. [2, 6]. Candidiasis, as an invasive candidal infection, is considered the most common fungal infectious disease around the world. In this regard, *C. albicans* and the NAC species including *Candida glabrata* and *Candida tropicalis,* rank first, second, and third, respectively, in association with global urinary tract infections (UTIs) [1, 3, 7].

In recent years, according to centers for disease control and prevention (CDC) reports [6], candidiasis infections caused by *Candida auris* have considerably risen up. Due to this knowledge, the results obtained from a study done by Meghan Lyman et al. in the United States of America (USA) show a significant increase in clinical cases in association with *C. auris*. They found a noticeable annual increase from 44 to 95% between 2019 and 2021 in the USA [8]. Totally, *C. auris* has been recognized as a progressive multidrug-resistant (MDR) candidal pathotype that can easily be distributed in public health centers and may lead to cause severe candidiasis in individuals [6]. The echinocandins-resistant strains of *C. auris* have been three-folded during 2 years from 2019 to 2021 [8].

In parallel with bacterial MDR features, the fungal MDR feature is a global public health concern that is highly growing up [5, 9]. Due to this fact, investigation in association with antifungal resistance molecular mechanisms in candidal infections may be a good option to control this group of invasive fungal infections.

2. Genomic characteristics and antifungal resistance feature

Genomic plasticity in eukaryotic opportunistic pathogens of fungi, including *Candida* spp., is known as a unique advantage that makes them adaptable to their environmental factors. Acquiring antifungal drug resistance feature is a considerable item in the field. In this regard, chromosomal rearrangement, aneuploidies, and the loss of heterozygosity, which are known as important genomic alterations, affect a versatile of fungal structures e.g., overexpression of efflux pumps and alterations in drug targets, that are involved in antifungal drug resistance feature in fungal pathogens [4, 10, 11].

3. A general view on antifungal drug resistance mechanisms

As aforementioned, we are now aware of different types of antifungal drug resistant mechanisms. Azoles, as fungistatic compounds, are one of the most common antifungal drugs which are composed of five-membered heterocycles and are categorized into two main groups of imidazole and triazole. Tioconazole, ketoconazole, clotrimazole, miconazole, econazole bear two nitrogen in their azole ring and due to this fact, they belong to imidazole group. On the other hand, the azoles of posaconazole, itraconazole, isavuconazole, fluconazole, and voriconazole are members of triazole group and bear three nitrogen in their azole ring. These antifungal drugs are administered to treat candidal infections or to prevent them. The target molecule of azole drugs is the 14α-demethylase enzyme, which plays a pivotal role in the fungal ergosterol biosynthesis pathway [3, 12–14]. Allylamines, morpholines, and polyenes are other classes of antifungal drugs that target other enzymes involved in the ergosterol biosynthesis pathway [3].

The fungicide antifungal drugs of echinocandins, such as, anidulafungin, caspofungin, and micafungin, inhibit the fungal cell wall biosynthesis by targeting the pivotal enzyme complex of β-1,3 glucan synthase [15–17].

Inhibition of the nucleic acid biosynthesis pathway is another target for some antifungal drugs, such as 5-Flucytosine (5FC). This antifungal drug is capable of inactivating the enzyme thymidylate synthase, which plays a pivotal role in the fungal biosynthesis pathway [18].

In accordance with the importance of effective treating procedures and the presence of different antifungals and the rise of antifungal drug resistance feature, it is necessary to apply new antifungal drugs or new strategies to replace current antifungal drug therapeutics.

Acknowledgements

The author has special thanks to Ms. Antonija Grgeč, the Publishing Process Manager of this project for her sincere full support and kind help.

Author contribution

The author has read and approved the latest version of the chapter.

Conflict of interest

The author declares no conflicts of interest.

Author details

Payam Behzadi
Department of Microbiology, Shahr-e-Qods Branch, Islamic Azad University, Tehran, Iran

*Address all correspondence to: behzadipayam@yahoo.com

References

[1] Behzadi P, Behzadi E, Ranjbar R. Urinary tract infections and *Candida albicans*. Central European Journal of Urology. 2015;**68**(1):96

[2] Behzadi P, Behzadi E. Modern Medical Mycology and Opportunistic Pathogenic Yeasts. Tehran: Persian Science & Research Publisher; 2011

[3] Bhattacharya S, Sae-Tia S, Fries BC. Candidiasis and mechanisms of antifungal resistance. Antibiotics. 2020;**9**(6):312

[4] Lee Y, Puumala E, Robbins N, Cowen LE. Antifungal drug resistance: Molecular mechanisms in *Candida albicans* and beyond. Chemical Reviews. 2020;**121**(6):3390-3411

[5] Czajka KM, Venkataraman K, Brabant-Kirwan D, Santi SA, Verschoor C, Appanna VD, et al. Molecular mechanisms associated with antifungal resistance in pathogenic Candida species. Cells. 2023;**12**(22):2655

[6] CDC. Candidiasis: CDC; 2022. Updated 2022. Available from: https://www.cdc.gov/fungal/diseases/candidiasis/index.html.

[7] Pfaller MA, Diekema D. Epidemiology of invasive candidiasis: A persistent public health problem. Clinical Microbiology Reviews. 2007;**20**(1):133-163

[8] Lyman M, Forsberg K, Sexton DJ, Chow NA, Lockhart SR, Jackson BR, et al. Worsening spread of Candida auris in the United States, 2019 to 2021. Annals of Internal Medicine. 2023;**176**(4):489-495

[9] Algammal A, Hetta HF, Mabrok M, Behzadi P. Emerging multidrug-resistant bacterial pathogens "superbugs": A rising public health threat. Frontiers in Microbiology. 2023;**14**:1135614

[10] Selmecki A, Forche A, Berman J. Genomic plasticity of the human fungal pathogen Candida albicans. Eukaryotic Cell. 2010;**9**(7):991-1008

[11] Chen G, Rubinstein B, Li R. Whole chromosome aneuploidy: Big mutations drive adaptation by phenotypic leap. BioEssays. 2012;**34**(10):893-900

[12] Yasu T, Konuma T, Kuroda S, Takahashi S, Tojo A. Effect of cumulative intravenous voriconazole dose on renal function in hematological patients. Antimicrobial Agents and Chemotherapy. 2018;**62**(9):1-4. DOI: 10.1128/aac00507-18

[13] Jenks JD, Salzer HJ, Prattes J, Krause R, Buchheidt D, Hoenigl M. Spotlight on isavuconazole in the treatment of invasive aspergillosis and mucormycosis: Design, development, and place in therapy. Drug Design, Development and Therapy. 2018;**12**:1033-1044

[14] Veen M, Stahl U, Lang C. Combined overexpression of genes of the ergosterol biosynthetic pathway leads to accumulation of sterols in *Saccharomyces cerevisiae*. FEMS Yeast Research. 2003;**4**(1):87-95

[15] Popolo L, Gualtieri T, Ragni E. The yeast cell-wall salvage pathway. Sabouraudia. 2001;**39**(1):111-121

[16] Perlin DS. Current perspectives on echinocandin class drugs. Future Microbiology. 2011;**6**(4):441-457

[17] Douglas C. Fungal β (1, 3)-D-glucan synthesis. Sabouraudia. 2001;**39**(1):55-66

[18] Vermes A, Guchelaar H-J, Dankert J. Flucytosine: A review of its pharmacology, clinical indications, pharmacokinetics, toxicity and drug interactions. Journal of Antimicrobial Chemotherapy. 2000;**46**(2):171-179

Section 2

Pathogenesis and Treatment

Chapter 2

Candida albicans: Pathogenesis and Secretory Pathways

Pia Afzelius, Charalampos Proestos and Payam Behzadi

Abstract

Candida albicans is a member of the human host's microbiome composition; therefore, it is recognized as a portion of the human host body's normal flora in a homeostasis condition. However, when the host develops an abnormal condition, e.g., immune deficiency, *C. albicans* acts as an opportunistic pathogen. *C. albicans* has an effective arsenal of a wide range of virulence factors. Due to this knowledge, the enzymes construct a significant portion of substantial fungal virulence factors, which are made of proteins and play an essential role in fungal invasion, fungal-hyphal growth, and biofilm formation. An active secreted protein should be processed via the fungal secretion system, such as the endoplasmic reticulum (ER) and/or Golgi apparatus (GA). In other words, an active protein that acts as a fungal virulence factor should undergo several vital and pivotal maturation processes, including glycosylation and folding. In this chapter, we have a rigorous look at these processes, which directly determine the pathogenesis of *C. albicans*.

Keywords: *Candida albicans*, pathogenesis, secretory pathways, glycosylation, virulence factors

1. Introduction

Fungi, including *Candida albicans* (*C. albicans*), as significant members of eukaryotes, can adapt to different environmental factors. Their flexible ability to adapt to other conditions is associated with vast metabolic pathways, morphogenetic characteristics, and life cycle diversities detected in fungal populations, e.g., *C. albicans*. Based on the reported results from previous investigations, the eukaryotic kingdom of fungi is estimated to possess 1.5 to 5 million species. The genome size of fungal species amazingly differs between 2 and 180 million nucleotides, and the proteome size of fungal species seems to range from 2 to 35 thousand [1, 2]. Although there is a wide range of fungal species, only a few fungi are known as primary or opportunistic pathogens. Among these pathogenic fungi, *Candida* spp., e.g., *C. albicans*, *C. auris, C. glabrata*, and *C. tropicalis* are identified as important fungal etiologic agents of human infectious diseases such as urogenital infections (vulvovaginal candidiasis, candidal balanitis), Candida onychomycosis, oropharyngeal candidiasis, skin candidiasis, and systemic candidiasis [2–8]. We know the human host is armed with many antifungal immune responses and signaling pathways; however, *C. albicans* also recruits its virulence factors to effectively oppose

IntechOpen

the human host defense system. *C. albicans,* as a dimorphic fungus, can adapt to the human host temperature, so it grows in its adhesive and invasive filamentous form. The filamentous form of *C. albicans* is the fungal invasive form that makes it capable of taking up nutrients from the human host body, charging its effective growth and progression, and escaping the human host immune system. Furthermore, several antifungal drug-resistant strains can easily resist antifungal therapeutics [2, 8]. Due to this knowledge, we will closely examine *C. albicans'* pathogenesis and secretory pathways.

2. Pan-genome of *Candida albicans*

In comparative genomic analyses, both eukaryotes and prokaryotes possess genomic pools composed of core- and accessory genomes. Usually, the core genome comprises those genes (housekeeping genes) that contribute to essential life activities, including reproduction, metabolism, cell division, virulence, and pathogenesis [9, 10]. On the other hand, the accessory (flexible, dispensable, and adaptive) genome contains genes that participate in specific functions, e.g., antibiotic resistance, specific metabolic pathways, and particular virulence, for the cell adaptation to its environment [9, 10]. The accessory genes are not present in all genomes but are usually detectable in ≥2 genomes. Hence, the genomic plasticity of the organisms is directly associated with mobile genetic elements [9–13]. Evolutionary biology studies depict two groups of genes, including analogous and homologous genes. The comparable genes appear through an independent converged evolutionary process, while the

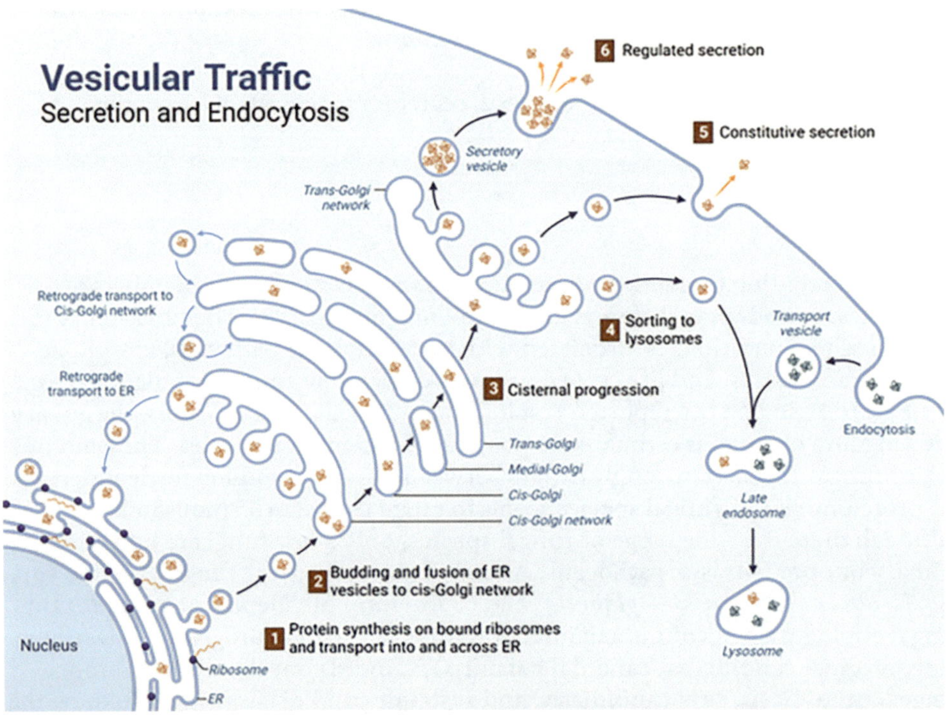

Figure 1.
The secretory pathway and the glycosylation processing including ER and GA (biorender.com).

homologous genes appear through an effective evolutionary process with identical origination from a similar ancestor. Furthermore, homologous genes are classified into two groups: paralogous genes, the outcome of the mutation feature, and orthologous genes – the outcome of evolutionary speciation [9, 10]. The results show that *C. albicans* is usually a diploid-genome yeast with 6189 genes in its pan-genomic pool. Six thousand sixty-nine genes constitute the core genomic pool. The 120 genes left form the flexible genome. The genomic investigations depict a close similarity (>80%) in nucleotide level among 5363 orthologous genes, which are shared between *C. albicans* and *C. dubliniensis* (a non-*Candida albicans* Candida (NCAC)) [14]. In this regard, it is estimated that >200 genes contribute to the trafficking of proteins within a limited secretory pathway of *C. albicans* (between different interior sections of the cell and the exterior cell surface). It does not include the proteins involved in post-translational modifications, protein folding, quality control, and those situated in the endoplasmic reticulum (ER) and Golgi apparatus (GA) (**Figure 1**). According to comparative genomic investigations, the secretory machinery constitution is conserved in eukaryotic cells, e.g., *C. albicans*. Moreover, the introns are detectable in only 8% of the genes in the secretory system [15–21].

3. Translocation

The secretory pathway fully mediates the virulence and the pathogenesis of pathogenic fungi like *C. albicans*. The protein secretion system participates in superficial adhesin secretion, immune system interacting proteins production, hydrolytic enzymes expression, phenotypic switching proteins secretion, and yeast-hypha transfigurative protein expression determines the capability, functionality, and dynamics of a cell [8, 15, 21]. The expressed proteins are initially inactive and should be activated. Hence, the biosynthesized ribosomal proteins should get the related modifications (such as glycosylation) and folding within the ER and then get packaged in the GA (**Figure 1**) [21].

4. Glycosylation

The glycosylation process begins with the quality control of a protein within the ER, which is the first section of the secretory pathway to check and mature the related proteins that are supposed to be glycosylated. On the other hand, the GA has been recognized as the leading center for glycosylation [22]. Indeed, the GA, recognized as the central hub of the cellular secretory machinery system, is made of different cisternae comprising the *cis*-Golgi network, *cis*, *medial*, *trans,* and *trans*-Golgi network with their topological characteristics and structures (**Figure 1**). Protein molecules get post-translational modifications within the GA cisternae and then depart to their final destination. The GA trafficking and homeostasis are directly associated with the vesicular trafficking machinery system (VTMS). The VTMS comprises tethers, small GTPase enzymes, soluble N-ethylmaleimide sensitive factor attachment protein receptors (SNAREs), and vesicular coats [23, 24]. The secreted and cell-surface proteins contribute to continuous and coordinated signaling between the cells within a multicellular organism. These proteins undergo post-translational modifications or glycosylation for the most to bear branched sugar polymers of the glycans with covalent bonds. The reported records show that glycome is involved in various biological activities, e.g., adhesion, protein folding, migration, cell stability, intracellular communication, and host-pathogen interactions. Depending on glycans' attachment to amino acids' hydroxyl group or amide group, two main types of glycoproteins including *O*-linked (attached glycans to threonines, serines, or hydroxylysines subsets)- and *N*-linked (attached glycans to asparagine residues; e.g., Asn-X(X is any amino acid excluding proline)-Ser/Thr) glycoproteins are recognized [25–28]. In addition, the attachment of glycosylphosphatidylinositol (GPI) to the cell wall and cell membrane proteins is known as post-translational modification, too. In other words, the GPI molecules anchor the cell wall and cell membrane proteins through covalent bonds. The biosynthetic pathway of GPI is a conserved metabolic pathway that occurs through several phases [28]. The GPI-anchored proteins support eukaryotes' growth and viability and are simultaneously critical factors of pathogenicity and virulence in eukaryotic pathogens like *C. albicans*. The central portion of the plasma membrane and dynamic structure of the cell wall in fungi such as *C. albicans* is formed by glycoproteins. Hence, the permeability, flexibility, plasticity, and suitable molecular scaffold in strong and impenetrable fungal cell walls are directly associated with glycans in the form of glycoproteins. According to previous studies, we now know that glycoproteins are pivotal biomolecules that contribute to different biological activities and functionalities. This feature results in effective morphogenesis, viability, and cell stability [27–30]. The structure and composition of the dynamic organelle of the fungal cell wall continuously interact and interchange with environmental factors and stresses [30]. That is why the fungal cell wall in pathogenic fungi can trigger the human host immune system and make the fungal cell capable of escaping from both innate and adaptive immune responses [31]. As previous investigations show, 20% (1200/6000 genes) of the genomic pool in *Saccharomyces cerevisiae* participates in the cell wall biosynthesis pathway [32]. *In toto*, the cell wall in fungi has a similar structure and composition because of its role and function. As mentioned earlier, the cell wall interacts with various peripheral factors, such as immune biomolecules in the human host. This layered organelle is supported by a conserved skeletal structure composed of a core section formed by glucan (branched ß-(1,3) with covalent linkages), interchain (3–4%), and chitin. Moreover, interchain hydrogen bonds between chitin and glucan result in microfilaments that cover the cell [30]. The branched glucan is linked to different biomolecules of proteins and or polysaccharides. The composition of proteins and polysaccharides may differ from one species to another among fungal populations [30]. ß-(1,3) and ß-(1,6) glycosidic bonds are identifiable within the linear molecules of D-glucose. The ß-(1,3) glucan contributes to the helical backbone, and the ß-(1,6) glucan is involved in branching structures through cross-linking with molecules of mannoproteins and chitins. This feature is supported by the GPI anchor attached to ß-(1,3) glucan [33].

Although glucan (α-(1,3)) is a practical construction in fungal cell wall structure and is associated with human fungal pathogens, it is absent in the cell wall structure of *C. albicans* and *S. cerevisiae* yeasts [30]. Because of fewer cell wall layers in the bud scar position, the yeast cell wall organelle encompasses a thinner diameter from the outside. Therefore, the inner side of the cell wall has been constructed by glucan (ß-(1,3)) and chitin composition [34, 35]. The fungal outer skeletal layers are very varied compared with the cell wall's inner layers. In both *C. albicans* and *S. cerevisiae*, the inner cell wall is entirely covered by a solid outer cell wall. A significant amount of mannosylated glycoproteins enriches the outer cell wall. The mannosylation process (recruitment of guanosine diphosphate (GDP)-mannose to create α- and ß-linked oligo mannosyl) is achieved via mannosyltransferase enzymes in *C. albicans* and *S. cerevisiae* [30, 36].

By recorded reports, a portion of the cell wall dry weight in *C. albicans* belongs to chitin molecules (up to ~2%), ß-(1,6) glucan (up to ~20%), and ß-(1,3) glucan [37, 38].

5. Protein glycosylation pathways

As aforementioned, the cell wall biosynthetic pathways in *C. albicans* are effective points of view in human-pathogen interactions because the glycosylated proteins and other fungal cell wall compositions (**Figure 2**), including structural polysaccharides such as chitin, chitosan, glucans, and *O*-, *N*-, and GPI-linked glycoproteins interact directly or indirectly with human host immune system. These fungal molecules are significant targets in producing new antifungal agents and immunotherapy methodologies [28, 39–42].

The biosynthetic pathway of *O*-linked glycosylation may produce and assemble linear oligosaccharides made of up to seven α-1,2-linked mannose residues. Although the feature of *O*-glycosylation is achieved within the GA [43], the ER lumen is where the attachment of α-linked mannose residues to threonine/serine residues takes place [44]. This process begins within the ER through the contribution of Dolichol (Dol)-P-Man, which acts as a sugar resource (**Figure 3**). The presence of protein mannosyltransferases achieves the sugar donation by Dol-P-Man. Protein mannosyltransferase enzymes are encoded by the gene family of *PMT1*, *PMT3*, *PMT4*, *PMT5*, and *PMT6* [45–47].

Indeed, Dolichol, composed of isoprene units, contributes to protein glycosylation modifications as a lipidic portion of the intermediates. The oligosaccharide of Dol-PP-$GlcNAc_2Man_5$ is produced by a combination of the sugar of mannose (Man) and *N*-acetyl-D-glucosamine (GlcNAc). In this biosynthetic pathway, GDP-Man and UDP-GlcNAc act as donor substrates or sugar donors [48–50].

The glycosylated proteins within the ER lumen move to GA to complete the glycosylation process. In this regard, the newly arrived glycoproteins into the Golgi complex undergo a new glycosylation process in which further mannose residues are linked. To catalyze this process, the Golgi-related α-1,2-mannosyltransferase enzymes -known as

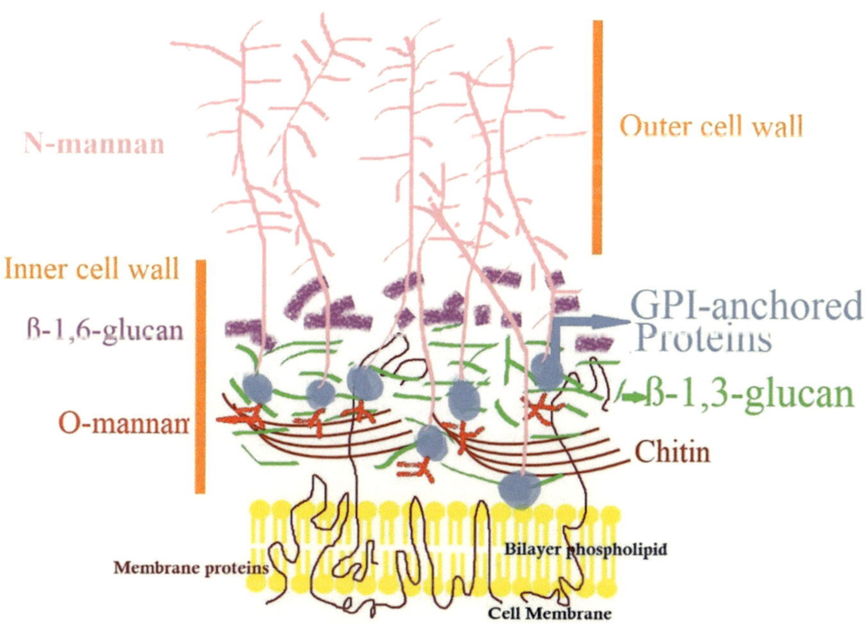

Figure 2.
The cell wall composition, structure, and the virulence factors associated with the pathogenesis in C. albicans.

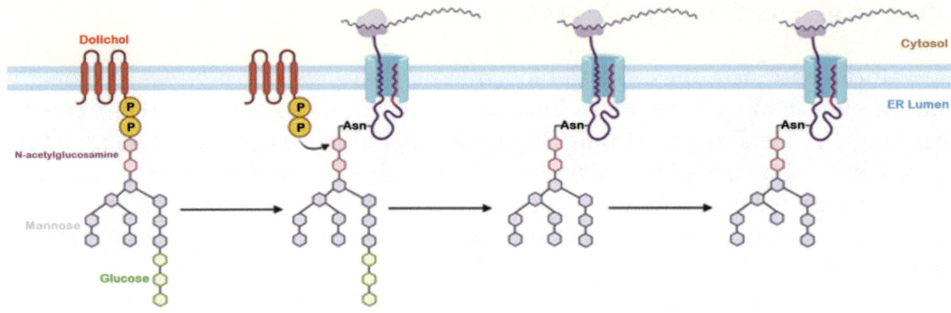

Figure 3.
Protein glycosylation in the endoplasmic reticulum (biorender.com).

GDP-mannose-dependent mannosyltransferases – contribute to this catalytic reaction. The genes of *MNT1* and *MNT2* encode the Golgi-located α-1,2-mannosyltransferase enzymes. The product of the *MNT1* gene (Mnt1) is involved in adding the second mannose residue, while the product of the *MNT2* gene (Mnt2) participates in the attachment of the third mannose residue to the *O*-linked glycan molecules. Both Mnt1 and Mnt2 are recognized as fungal virulence elements. The phosphomannosylation of *O*-linked glycans may be occurred by the Mnt3 and Mnt5 enzymes [46, 51, 52].

The fungal *N*-linked glycosylation pathway in *C. albicans* is known as an effective process because the initial phases of *N*-linked protein glycosylation are recognized as conserved eukaryotic processes that are observed in different eukaryotic cells from fungi to plants and from mammals to protozoa. The biosynthesis of *N*-linked glycans contains a collection of enzymatic reactions and modifications that should occur in ER and GA. In this regard, the essential enzymes of glycosyltransferases and glycosidases have pivotal keys in this biosynthetic pathway. In the first step, the ER (rough ER (RER))-located glycosyltransferase enzymes contribute to an assemblage of an oligosaccharide molecule upon a targeted isoprenoid lipid. In the second step, the ER-located glycosidase enzymes and Golgi-located glycosyltransferase enzymes catalyze additional modifications relating to *N*-linked glycan molecules [28, 53]. Glycosidase enzymes are glycoside hydrolyses that contribute to glycosidic bond hydrolysis in glycosides. These glycoside molecules are detectable in various substances, such as glycoproteins, fungi, and other organisms. The Carbohydrate-Active EnZyme database http://www.cazy.org/) (December 4, 2023) present 187 families of glycoside hydrolase enzymes (http://www.cazy.org/Glycoside-Hydrolases.html), 117 families relating to glycosyltransferases (http://www.cazy.org/GlycosylTransferases.html), 43 families in association with polysaccharide lyase enzymes (http://www.cazy.org/Polysaccharide-Lyases.html), 20 families regarding carbohydrate esterases (http://www.cazy.org/Carbohydrate-Esterases.html), and 17 families associated with auxiliary activities (http://www.cazy.org/Auxiliary-Activities.html) [54, 55].

6. Conclusion

The secretory system of *C. albicans* involves many fungal cell structures and functions. In this regard, many structural compositions and activities are identified as a double-edged sword. However, the cell wall compositions are recognized as a pathogenic arsenal and virulence factor in medical mycology. For instance, glucans participate in *C. albicans* biofilm formation, and the production of these cell wall materials may be promoted during this feature. Formation of biofilm may increase the feature of antifungal drug resistance, and this unfavored occurrence is known as a big challenge in the public healthcare system and medicine.

Acknowledgements

The authors have special thanks to IntechOpen publisher for the kind invitation. We also appreciate Antonija Grgec, the Publishing Process Manager of the present book project, for her brilliant support. **Figures 1** and **3** are directly taken from biorender.com. Hence, the authors are obliged to biorender.com, too.

Author contribution

The authors have contributed to the present chapter. All the authors have read and approved the latest version of the chapter.

Conflict of interest

The authors declare no conflicts of interest.

Author details

Pia Afzelius[1], Charalampos Proestos[2] and Payam Behzadi[3]*

1 Department of Clinical Physiology and Nuclear Medicine Odense, Odense University Hospital, Denmark

2 Laboratory of Food Chemistry, Department of Chemistry, National and Kapodistrian University of Athens Zografou, Athens, Greece

3 Department of Microbiology, Shahr-e-Qods Branch, Islamic Azad University, Tehran, Iran

*Address all correspondence to: behzadipayam@yahoo.com

References

[1] Choi J, Kim S-H. A genome tree of life for the fungi kingdom. National Academy of Sciences of the United States of America. 2017;**114**(35):9391-9396

[2] Lopes JP, Lionakis MS. Pathogenesis and virulence of *Candida albicans*. Virulence. 2022;**13**(1):89-121

[3] Behzadi P, Behzadi E, Ranjbar R. Urinary tract infections and *Candida albicans*. Central European Journal of Urology. 2015;**68**(1):96-101

[4] Behzadi P, Behzadi E, Pawlak-Adamska EA. Urinary tract infections (UTIs) or genital tract infections (GTIs)? It's the diagnostics that count. GMS Hygiene and Infection Control. 2019;**14**:1-12

[5] Behzadi P, Behzadi E. The microbial agents of urinary tract infections at central laboratory of Dr. Shariati hospital, Tehran, Iran. Turk Klin Tip Bilim. 2008;**28**(4):445-449

[6] Behzadi P, Behzadi E, Yazdanbod H, Aghapour R, Cheshmeh MA, Omran DS. Urinary tract infections associated with *Candida albicans*. Maedica. 2010;**5**(4):277-279

[7] Behzadi P, Behzadi E. Evaluation of UVB light efficacy for inducing apoptosis in *Candida albicans* cultures. Roumanian Archives of Microbiology and Immunology. 2012;**71**(1):39-42

[8] Behzadi P, Behzadi E. Modern Medical Mycology and Opportunistic Pathogenic Yeasts. Tehran: Persian Science & Research Publisher; 2011

[9] Costa SS, Guimarães LC, Silva A, Soares SC, Baraúna RA. First steps in the analysis of prokaryotic pan-genomes. Bioinformatics and Biology Insights. 2020;**14**:1177932220938064

[10] Vernikos G, Medini D, Riley DR, Tettelin H. Ten years of pan-genome analyses. Current Opinion in Microbiology. 2015;**23**:148-154

[11] Sarshar M, Behzadi P, Ambrosi C, Zagaglia C, Palamara AT, Scribano D. FimH and anti-adhesive therapeutics: A disarming strategy against uropathogens. Antibiotics. 2020;**9**(7):397

[12] Behzadi P. Uropathogenic Escherichia Coli and Fimbrial Adhesins Virulome. Urinary Tract Infection: The Result of the Strength of the Pathogen, or the Weakness of the Host. Croatia: InTechOpen; 2018. pp. 65-83

[13] Behzadi P, Behzadi E. Uropathogenic Escherichia coli: An ideal resource for DNA microarray probe designing. In: Bioinformatics and Biomedical Engineering: 5th International Work-Conference, IWBBIO 2017, Granada, Spain, April 26-28, 2017, Proceedings, Part II 5. Switzerland: Springer; 2017

[14] Richard G-F. Eukaryotic pangenomes. In: The Pangenome: Diversity, Dynamics and Evolution of Genomes. Cham (CH): Springer; 2020. pp. 253-291

[15] Fonzi WA. The protein secretory pathway of *Candida albicans*. Mycoses. 2009;**52**(4):291-303

[16] Braun BR, van Het Hoog M, d'Enfert C, Martchenko M, Dungan J, Kuo A, et al. A human-curated annotation of the *Candida albicans* genome. PLoS Genetics. 2005;**1**(1):e1

[17] Gupta GD, Heath IB. Predicting the distribution, conservation, and functions

of SNAREs and related proteins in fungi. Fungal Genetics and Biology. 2002;**36**(1):1-21

[18] Swennen D, Beckerich J-M. Yarrowia lipolytica vesicle-mediated protein transport pathways. BMC Evolutionary Biology. 2007;**7**:1-19

[19] Bock JB, Matern HT, Peden AA, Scheller RH. A genomic perspective on membrane compartment organization. Nature. 2001;**409**(6822):839-841

[20] Mitrovich QM, Tuch BB, Guthrie C, Johnson AD. Computational and experimental approaches double the number of known introns in the pathogenic yeast *Candida albicans*. Genome Research. 2007;**17**(4):492-502

[21] Rollenhagen C, Mamtani S, Ma D, Dixit R, Eszterhas S, Lee SA. The role of secretory pathways in *Candida albicans* pathogenesis. Journal of Fungi. 2020;**6**(1):26

[22] Kim C-H, Kim C-H. N-glycan and O-glycan glycosylation in eukaryotes. In: Ganglioside Biochemistry. Singapore: Springer; 2020. pp. 15-34

[23] D'Souza Z, Sumya FT, Khakurel A, Lupashin V. Getting sugar coating right! The role of the golgi trafficking machinery in glycosylation. Cells. 2021;**10**(12):3275

[24] Yoon T-Y, Munson M. SNARE complex assembly and disassembly. Current Biology. 2018;**28**(8):R397-R401

[25] Bard F, Chia J. Cracking the glycome encoder: Signaling, trafficking, and glycosylation. Trends in Cell Biology. 2016;**26**(5):379-388

[26] Lin B, Qing X, Liao J, Zhuo K. Role of protein glycosylation in host-pathogen interaction. Cells. 2020;**9**(4):1022

[27] Lin G-Y, Chang C-F, Lan C-Y. The interaction between carbohydrates and the antimicrobial peptide P-113Tri is involved in the killing of *Candida albicans*. Microorganisms. 2020;**8**(2):299

[28] Gómez-Gaviria M, Vargas-Macías AP, García-Carnero LC, Martínez-Duncker I, Mora-Montes HM. Role of protein glycosylation in interactions of medically relevant fungi with the host. Journal of Fungi. 2021;**7**(10):875

[29] Yadav U, Khan MA. Targeting the GPI biosynthetic pathway. Pathogens and Global Health. 2018;**112**(3):115-122

[30] Gow NA, Latge J-P, Munro CA. The fungal cell wall: Structure, biosynthesis, and function. Microbiology Spectrum. 2017;**5**(3)

[31] Erwig LP, Gow NA. Interactions of fungal pathogens with phagocytes. Nature Reviews Microbiology. 2016;**14**(3):163-176

[32] de Groot PW, Ruiz C, Vázquez de Aldana CR, Dueñas E, Cid VJ, Del Rey F, et al. A genomic approach for the identification and classification of genes involved in cell wall formation and its regulation in *Saccharomyces cerevisiae*. Comparative and Functional Genomics. 2001;**2**(3):124-142

[33] Reyna-Beltrán E, Isaac Bazán Méndez C, Iranzo M, Mormeneo S, Pedro L-AJ. The cell wall of Candida albicans: A proteomics view. In: Candida albicans. Vol. 12. London, United Kingdom (UK): IntechOpen; 2019. pp. 71-92

[34] Wheeler RT, Kombe D, Agarwala SD, Fink GR. Dynamic, morphotype-specific *Candida albicans* β-glucan exposure during infection and drug treatment. PLoS Pathogens. 2008;**4**(12):e1000227

[35] Kapteyn J, Hoyer L, Hecht J, Müller W, Andel A, Verkleij A, et al.

The cell wall architecture of *Candida albicans* wild-type cells and cell wall-defective mutants. Molecular Microbiology. 2000;**35**(3):601-611

[36] Hall RA, Gow NA. Mannosylation in *Candida albicans*: Role in cell wall function and immune recognition. Molecular Microbiology. 2013;**90**(6):1147-1161

[37] Ruiz-Herrera J, Victoria Elorza M, Valentín E, Sentandreu R. Molecular organization of the cell wall of *Candida albicans* and its relation to pathogenicity. FEMS Yeast Research. 2006;**6**(1):14-29

[38] Latgé JP. The cell wall: A carbohydrate Armour for the fungal cell. Molecular Microbiology. 2007;**66**(2):279-290

[39] Lenardon MD, Sood P, Dorfmueller HC, Brown AJ, Gow NA. Scalar nanostructure of the *Candida albicans* cell wall; a molecular, cellular and ultrastructural analysis and interpretation. The Cell Surface. 2020;**6**:100047

[40] Gow NA, Van De Veerdonk FL, Brown AJ, Netea MG. *Candida albicans* morphogenesis and host defence: Discriminating invasion from colonization. Nature Reviews Microbiology. 2012;**10**(2):112-122

[41] Zhou Y, Cheng L, Lei YL, Ren B, Zhou X. The interactions between *Candida albicans* and mucosal immunity. Frontiers in Microbiology. 2021;**12**:652725

[42] Gow NA, Hube B. Importance of the *Candida albicans* cell wall during commensalism and infection. Current Opinion in Microbiology. 2012;**15**(4):406-412

[43] Herscovics A, Orlean P. Glycoprotein biosynthesis in yeast. The FASEB Journal. 1993;**7**(6):540-550

[44] Lehle L, Strahl S, Tanner W. Protein glycosylation, conserved from yeast to man: A model organism helps elucidate congenital human diseases. Angewandte Chemie International Edition. 2006;**45**(41):6802-6818

[45] Martínez-Duncker I, Díaz-Jímenez DF, Mora-Montes HM. Comparative analysis of protein glycosylation pathways in humans and the fungal pathogen *Candida albicans*. International Journal of Microbiology. 2014;**2014**:267497

[46] Díaz-Jiménez DF, Mora-Montes HM, Hernández-Cervantes A, Luna-Arias JP, Gow NA, Flores-Carreón A. Biochemical characterization of recombinant *Candida albicans* mannosyltransferases Mnt1, Mnt2 and Mnt5 reveals new functions in O-and N-mannan biosynthesis. Biochemical and Biophysical Research Communications. 2012;**419**(1):77-82

[47] Goto M. Protein O-glycosylation in fungi: Diverse structures and multiple functions. Bioscience, Biotechnology, and Biochemistry. 2007;**71**(6):1415-1427

[48] Cha J-H, Hong M, Cha C-J. Fungal β-glycosidase belonging to subfamily 4 of glycoside hydrolase family 30 with transglycosylation activity. Journal of Agricultural and Food Chemistry. 2021;**69**(50):15261-15267

[49] Cattò C, Corte L, Roscini L, Cardinali G, Villa F, Cappitelli F. Metabolomic and proteomic changes in *Candida albicans* biofilm in response to zosteric acid treatment. International Journal of Molecular Sciences. 2022;**23**(22):14067

[50] Rossow JA, Queiroz-Telles F, Caceres DH, Beer KD, Jackson BR, Pereira JG, et al. A one health approach to combatting *Sporothrix brasiliensis*: Narrative review of an emerging zoonotic

fungal pathogen in South America. Journal of Fungi. 2020;**6**(4):247

[51] Mora-Montes HM, Bates S, Netea MG, Castillo L, Buurman BA, et al. A multifunctional mannosyltransferase family in *Candida albicans* determines cell wall mannan structure and host-fungus interactions. Journal of Biological Chemistry. 2010;**285**(16):12087-12095

[52] Munro CA, Bates S, Buurman ET, Hughes HB, MacCallum DM, Bertram G, et al. Mnt1p and Mnt2p of *Candida albicans* are partially redundant α-1, 2-mannosyltransferases that participate in O-linked mannosylation and are required for adhesion and virulence. Journal of Biological Chemistry. 2005;**280**(2):1051-1060

[53] Ortiz-Ramírez JA, Cuéllar-Cruz M, Villagómez-Castro JC, López-Romero E. Fungal glycosidases in sporothrix species and *Candida albicans*. Journal of Fungi. 2023;**9**(9):919

[54] Divakar S, Divakar S. Glycosidases. In: Enzymatic Transformation. New Delhi: Springer; 2013. pp. 5-21

[55] Drula E, Garron M-L, Dogan S, Lombard V, Henrissat B, Terrapon N. The carbohydrate-active enzyme database: Functions and literature. Nucleic Acids Research. 2022;**50**(D1):D571-D5D7

Chapter 3

Invasive Candidiasis Due to *Candida albicans* and Its Treatment

Javier Aquiles Hidalgo Acosta, María Fernanda Calderón León, Nataly del Carmen Quisiguiña Jarrin, Paola Vanessa Solorzano Acosta, Mariuxi Vanessa Viteri Herrera, Silvio Paul Carlosama Ruiz, Brigitte Carolina Guerra Espinoza, Wendy Belén Iguasnia Guala, Jorge Eduardo Bejarano Macias and Anthony Guillermo Merino Estrella

Abstract

Invasive candidiasis secondary to *Candida albicans* should be highly suspected in patients exposed to the various risk factors that contribute to the affectation of this fungus, in order to provide early management of sepsis, through the use of antifungals in a timely manner, and to avoid the development of multiorgan failure. Diagnosis is fundamental and is based on laboratory studies, cultures, and risk scales; however, there are still limitations due to the fact that they do not have 100% sensitivity or specificity. Echinocandins remain the first line of treatment for patients with invasive candidiasis associated with *C. albicans*. Invasive candidiasis can affect any organ and increase mortality in adult and neonatal intensive care unit patients.

Keywords: invasive fungal infections, *Candida albicans*, diagnosis, treatment, candidiasis, invasive

1. Introduction

The importance of the chapter is justified by the need to know the current perspective on the epidemiology, diagnosis, and treatment of invasive candidiasis, caused by *Candida albicans*, to be able to recognize and treat severe complications such as fungal sepsis, which represents a high mortality, mainly in immunocompromised patients.

Invasive candidiasis is a serious infection, most frequently caused by the genus *Candida albicans*, and can manifest as sepsis, with multiorgan dysfunction and septic shock. *C. Albicans* accounts for 50% of all causes of fungal sepsis in the intensive care unit, with a mortality rate of between 40 and 70%, so its diagnosis and treatment are relevant. *C. albicans* belongs to the eumycetes and is an opportunistic pathogen, which is characterized by having a unicellular body, being a pseudomycelium [1].

C. albicans infection is pathogenic when there is a deterioration in immunity, with previous colonization, changes in the normal flora, bacterial translocation, or other factors associated with the deterioration of cellular immunity. After invading the mucous membranes, *Candida* proliferates; adheres, forming plaques; and then spreads through the vascular system, causing candidemia, which is defined as the presence of Candida in the blood [2, 3]. Candidemia causes T cell depletion and infects any organ, causing invasive candidiasis [4]. About 80% of *C. albicans* infections are associated with the formation of biofilms in different medical devices; the development of biofilms represents a greater systemic invasion and therefore a greater inflammatory response and resistance to antifungals [5].

C. albicans is the most frequently isolated germ in invasive candidiasis, associated with various risk factors, such as: the use of permanent medical devices, a prolonged hospital stay, and the use of antibiotics [6, 7]. It is classified into invasive candidiasis with candidemia, invasive candidiasis without candidemia, and candidemia alone [8].

The main risk factors for invasive candidiasis by *C. albicans* are age, mainly in preterm infants; HIV infection with CD4 < 200; use of corticosteroids, total parenteral nutrition; deep candidiasis; septic shock with multiorgan failure; invasive fungal infection in newborns [9]; central venous catheter transfusions [10]; previous colonization [10]; hematologic malignancies, chemotherapy [11]; and hospital-acquired intravascular infections.

There are differences in the predominance of germs in both patients admitted to adult and pediatric critical care units, so much so that there is a growing predominance of *C. no albicans* in pediatric ICUs, such as *C. parapsilosis* (43%) [12].

Invasive candidiasis can affect any organ or system, due to exposure to various factors such as: alterations of the intestinal mucosa, virulence factors of the fungus, and predisposition to biofilm formation [13].

Cerebral candidiasis is common in patients with primary or secondary immunodeficiencies; it is observed in the form of *C. albicans* meningoencephalitis [14].

Respiratory candidiasis presents in the form of bronchopulmonary candidiasis, represents a rare cause of pneumonia, and is associated with states of severe immunosuppression; if this is suspected, a fibrobronchoscopy with bronchoalveolar lavage can be performed for its diagnosis [15].

Renal candidiasis, can cause kidney damage in kidney transplant recipients; in these cases, it is observed in the isolates: *Candida no albicans, C. famata, C. tropicalis, C. parapsilosis, C. glabrata, and C. lusitaniae; however, Candida albicans* continues to be the most frequent cause of renal candidiasis [16, 17].

Severe urogenital candidiasis and vulvovaginal candidiasis can present in the form of abscesses, pelviperitonitis, emphysematous cystitis, emphysematous pyelonephritis in polymicrobial infections; are more frequent in patients with poorly controlled diabetes mellitus who are pregnant; and can transform into invasive candidiasis if adequate treatment is not carried out.

Fungemia in patients with hematological malignancies, chemotherapy, and neutropenia are the important risk factors for high mortality.

Blood cultures play an important role in the first hour of sepsis, although the sensitivity and specificity proven ranges between 21 and 71%. Other supportive diagnostic methods are beta-D-glucan and procalcitonin biomarkers, with favorable results in the exclusion of invasive candidiasis with a sensitivity of 98% and negative predictive value of 95%. Since 50% of cultures for invasive candidiasis are negative, they have suggested diagnostic tests such as mannan/antimannan, germ tube antibody para-*C. albicans*, 1,3-β-d-glucan, polymerase chain reaction, and T2Candida panel, which aid early diagnosis before blood culture results and are of great importance. They should be performed on all patients with suspected invasive candidiasis due to *C. albicans*, as they improve treatment performance [18, 19].

Other recommended studies are the echocardiogram, when candidiasis of cardiac origin is suspected with the presence of vegetation in the valves or hemodialysis catheters; ophthalmoscopy can also be performed to visualize ocular infection in patients with invasive candidiasis.

Once the diagnosis has been made with a positive culture, it is necessary to follow the blood cultures until they are negative, and it is recommended to continue the treatment for 14 days after the negative result [20], another score used is the Candida Score due to multifocal colonization by *Candida*; admission to the ICU for surgery, sepsis, and parenteral nutrition allow a diagnostic approach to be made and a risk score assigned in patients with suspected invasive candidiasis, which can be started early according to high, medium, or low risk.

Echinocandins are the first-line antifungals for the treatment of invasive candidiasis [21]. In recent years, an increase in resistance to fluconazole and echinocandins by *C. albicans* has been observed, which has generated an epidemiological change to multidrug-resistant germs or other types of non-albicans Candida; the de-escalation from an echinocandin to fluconazole can be performed when the germ is susceptible [22, 23].

Caspofungin is a fungicide against *C. albicans*, which belongs to the lipopeptides; its mechanism of action is inhibition of the synthesis of 1,3-beta-d-glucan of the cell wall; the loading dose is 70 mg followed by 50 mg daily or 70 mg each day. In patients with chronic kidney disease or hemodialysis, the same dose is considered; in patients with hepatic impairment, a decrease in its effect is observed.

Anidulafungin is an echinocandin used for the management of invasive candidiasis, with a loading dose of 200 mg and maintenance dose 100 mg daily; its effect is not affected by chronic kidney disease, and it is not necessary to adjust the dose in kidney disease, nor is it affected by liver failure; in the pediatric population, the dose (3 mg/kg on day 1, 1.5 mg/kg maintenance dose) has obtained good results, with success rates of 68.8% response to treatment in pediatric candidemia [24].

Micafungin is also effective for the management of invasive candidiasis at doses of 100 mg intravenously passed in 1 hour each day, with good penetration to the central nervous system for cerebral candidiasis [25, 26].

Another management that we fear to take into consideration in the event of invasive candidiasis is to remove all medical devices such as catheters, central venous catheters, and hemodialysis catheters [27].

The main objective of the chapter is to determine the current therapeutics of invasive candidiasis caused by *C. albicans*.

2. Methodology

A search was carried out in databases and medical journals of high prestige such as PubMed, Mendeley, IntechOpen, LILACS, and Latindex; as a search pattern, the research question was used; clear, precise, and concise articles that addressed the topic, published in the last 5 years, were included.

3. Invasive candidiasis from different aspects

Observational studies, randomized trials, clinical cases, guidelines, systematic reviews, meta-analyses, and consensus documents on the epidemiology, risk factors, and diagnosis of invasive candidiasis due *to Candida albicans* and its current treatment were obtained.

C. albicans is a frequent cause of hospital infection at the level of adult and neonatal intensive care. **Table 1** represents the types of locations such as esophageal and ophthalmic that can generate or be a consequence of candidemia or invasive candidiasis, risk factors for invasive candidiasis, and also as a frequent cause of sepsis and multiorgan failure. **Table 2** discusses studies with the percentage of isolation for

Author	Type of Candidiasis	*C. albicans*	Risk factor for *Candida albicans*
Robertson, et al. 2023	Esophageal candidiasis	88% of esophagitis are secondary to *C. albicans*	Age, HIV infection, and corticosteroid use correlate with candidal esophagitis.
Phongkhun, et al. 2023	Ocular Candidiasis and *Candida* Endophthalmitis in candidemia Patients	The presence of *C. albicans* was associated with *Candida* endophthalmitis	Total parenteral nutrition has been associated with C. *albicans* candidiasis and causes ocular candidiasis
McCarty, et al. 2023	Candidemia and invasive candidiasis	85% of cases presented with candidemia and 15% presented without candidemia	Hospital-acquired bloodstream infections in patients admitted to critical care units
Gonzalez-Lara, et al. 2020.	Invasive candidiasis	The most common causative agent is *C. albicans*	Profound candidiasis and septic shock with multiorgan failure.
Ferrando, et al. 2023	Neonatal invasive candidiasis	*Candida albicans* is the most common cause of invasive fungal disease in preterm and/or low-birth weight infants	Invasive fungal infection in newborns

Author: Javier Aquiles, Hidalgo Acosta.

Table 1.
Risk factors for invasive candidiasis caused by C. albicans.

Author	Invasive candidiasis by study region	Diagnosis
Okoye, et al. 2022	Invasive candidiasis in Africa	*C. albicans* 32.6% of cases
Wang, et al. 2022	Invasive candidiasis in critically ill patients in Anhui, China	*C. albicans* 41.49% of reports
Franco, 2021	Invasive candidiasis in Mexico and Spain	In the Spanish pediatrics population *C. albicans* 36%, Mexican pediatric patients *C. albicans* infections predominate (64%). In Spanish adult patients *C. albicans (40–75%).* In Mexican adult patients, *C. albicans* 62%.

Author: Javier Aquiles, Hidalgo Acosta.

Table 2.
Invasive candidiasis due to C. albicans *according to the study region and the percentage of* C. albicans *diagnoses.*

DOI: http://dx.doi.org/10.5772/intechopen.1004148

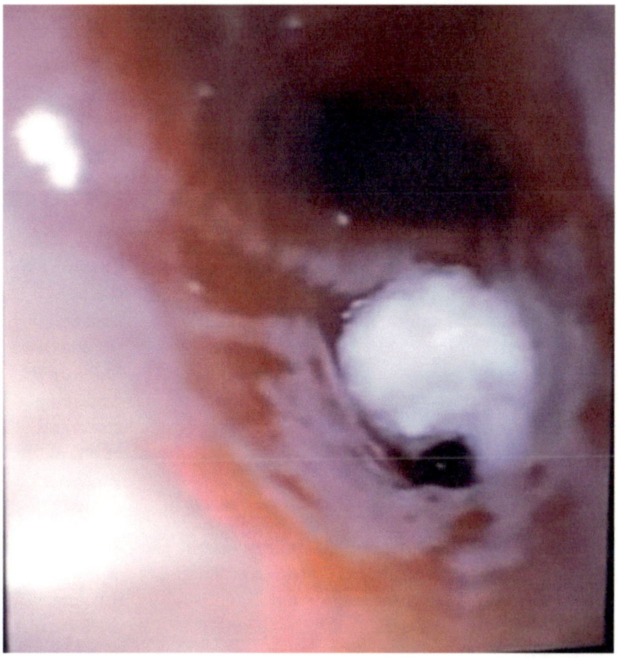

Figure 1.
Image of the tracheal lumen observed during a flexible diagnostic fibrobronchoscopy in a patient with invasive candidiasis of pulmonary focus; an exophytic white image inside the bronchus with a whitish tracheal mucosa with a tendency to bleed can be evidenced. Source: Dr. Javier Aquiles Hidalgo Acosta.

C. albicans in patients with invasive candidiasis according to the region of study, which presents different results due to different epidemiological aspects; Africa reported the lowest percentages of isolates, followed by Anhui in China, unlike Mexico and Spain with higher percentages of cultures for *C. albicans*. **Figure 1** shows an infection by an invasive candidiasis of pulmonary origin with changes in the appearance

Author	Intervention	Population	Dose	Results	Conclusions
Thompson, et al. 2023	Rezafungin versus caspofungin for the treatment of candidemia and invasive (ReSTORE)	≥18 years with systemic signs and mycological confirmation of candidemia or invasive candidiasis	Weekly intravenous rezafungin (400 mg at week 1, followed by 200 mg weekly, for a total of two to four doses) or intravenous caspofungin (loading dose of 70 mg on day 1). followed by 50 mg daily) for no more than 4 weeks.	(59%) of patients in the rezafungin group and (61%) of patients in the caspofungin group had an overall cure on day 14. Mortality (24%) in the rezafungin group and (21%) in caspofungin patients	Rezafungin was not inferior to caspofungin for overall cure at day 14 and all-cause mortality at 30 days.

Author	Intervention	Population	Dose	Results	Conclusions
Roilides, et al. 2019	Safety, Tolerability, and Efficacy of Anidulafungin in the Treatment of Invasive Candidiasis	Children 2 to <18 years of age	3 mg/kg on day 1, 1.5 mg/kg daily	All-cause mortality ranged from 8.2% to 14.3%	Anidulafungin as a treatment option for invasive candidiasis in children aged 2 to <18 years
Kim, et al. 2020	Caspofungin versus amphotericin B deoxycholate in the treatment of invasive candidiasis in neonates	Neonates and infants under 3 months of age	2 mg/kg caspofungin intravenously once daily or 1 mg/kg amphotericin B deoxycholate	The survival rate at 2 weeks after treatment was 71.0% in the caspofungin group and 68.8% in the amphotericin group	Amphotericin had more adverse effects with similar mortality
Auriti, et al. 2021	High-dose micafungin in neonates and young infants with invasive candidiasis	neonates and young infants with invasive candidiasis	micafungin at doses of 8 mg/kg	Resolution of infection was achieved in 86.7% of treated patients	Micafungin at a dose of 8 mg/kg daily is effective and well tolerated in neonates and young infants
Kullberg, et al. 2019	Isavuconazole versus caspofungin in the treatment of candidemia and other invasive Candida infections	Adult patients with candidemia or invasive candidiasis.	Isavuconazole (200 mg intravenously [IV] three times daily for 2 days, followed by 200 mg IV once daily or caspofungin 70 mg IV on day 1, followed by 50 mg IV [70 mg in patients >80 kg])	A successful overall response was observed in 60.3% of patients in the isavuconazole group and 71.1% in the caspofungin group	Caspofungin was superior as an initial empirical treatment
Spec, et al. 2019	Oral Ibrexafungerp After Initial Echinocandin-Based Therapy	Non-neutropenic patients with invasive candidiasis	Ibrexafungerp 750 mg versus standard of care	Similar favorable response rates across all ibrexafungerp groups: 86%	The estimated oral dose of ibrexafungerp to reach target exposure in subjects with invasive candidiasis is 750 mg daily. This dose was well tolerated and achieved a similar favorable overall response rate

Author	Intervention	Population	Dose	Results	Conclusions
Pappas, et al. 2023	Fosmanogepix, for the treatment of candidemia	Non-neutropenic adults. Participants with candidemia, defined as a positive blood culture for Candida spp.	1000 mg IV twice daily on day 1, followed by 600 mg IV maintenance once daily and optional switch to 700 mg orally once daily starting on day 4	Treatment success was 80% and survival at day 30 was 85%	Fosmanogepix may be a safe, well-tolerated, and effective treatment for non-neutropenic patients with candidemia

Author: Javier Aquiles, Hidalgo Acosta.

Table 3.
A current treatment of invasive candidiasis from randomized phase 2 and 3 clinical studies on the safety and efficacy of the different treatments.

of the tracheal mucosa; the mucosa is shown with a tendency to bleed and a white exophytic image with a result of pulmonary candidiasis, which proves that invasive candidiasis due *to Candida* can affect any organ or system when it occurs invasively. In some cases, invasive procedures are necessary for early diagnosis and treatment, and patients with risk factors must be highly suspicious.

Table 3 shows the current therapeutics from randomized trials on the treatment of invasive candidiasis. Echinocandins (caspofungin, anidulafungin, rezafungin, micafungin) are the most widely used first-line treatment with better results. New drugs (Fosmanogepix, ibrexafungerp) improve the possibility of administering oral doses, and other drugs already used such as amphotericin have also demonstrated their efficacy. As therapeutic options for the management of invasive candidiasis, new molecules have emerged for the treatment of this fungal sepsis [28–33].

4. Conclusions

Blood cultures do not have a specificity and sensitivity of 100% to predict the decision to start or withdraw antifungal treatment in the face of suspected invasive fungal infection, worse if it is an immunosuppressed patient whose clinical debut is atypical, so it is necessary to take advantage of the golden hour and use more effective diagnostic tests and the appropriate time, hand in hand, with the analysis of the risk and epidemiological factors corresponding to *Candida albicans*.

Previous colonization is one of the most important factors found for invasive candidiasis; among others, HIV, parenteral nutrition, bloodstream infections, sepsis, septic shock, multiorgan failure, and neonatal infection are very important factors to initiate empirical antifungal therapy and thus improve survival in patients with invasive candidiasis caused by *C. albicans.*

Obtaining blood culture samples in the golden 1st hour of sepsis in patients with risk factors for invasive candidiasis will allow early treatment to be initiated in populations with increased risk of invasive candidiasis. It is necessary to investigate the reason for the marked epidemiological changes that may be associated with various factors. Mexico presented the highest percentages of *C. albicans* followed by Spain, China, and Africa in patients with invasive candidiasis.

Acknowledgements

A special thanks to my mother, teacher Mrs. Juana Narcisa Acosta Alcívar, an example to follow in education in Ecuador, Abigucho, Claris, Lucciana, Gladys, This is done with full funding from the authors.

Conflict of interest

The authors declare no conflict of interest.

Appendices and nomenclature

C	*Candida*
HIV	human immunodeficiency virus
CD4	CD4 T lymphocytes
ICU	intensive care unit
EQUAL	quality of clinical candidemia management
IV	intravenous

Author details

Javier Aquiles Hidalgo Acosta[1*], María Fernanda Calderón León[2*], Nataly del Carmen Quisiguiña Jarrin[3*], Paola Vanessa Solorzano Acosta[4*], Mariuxi Vanessa Viteri Herrera[5*], Silvio Paul Carlosama Ruiz[6*], Brigitte Carolina Guerra Espinoza[7*], Wendy Belén Iguasnia Guala[8*], Jorge Eduardo Bejarano Macias[9*] and Anthony Guillermo Merino Estrella[10*]

1 Teodoro Maldonado Carbo Hospital, Guayaquil, Ecuador

2 University Hospital, Guayaquil, Ecuador

3 Metropolitan Medical Clinic Hospital, Riobamba, Ecuador

4 Machala General Hospital, Ecuadorian Institute of Social Security and Medical, Private University of Specialties Espíritu Santo, Samborondón, Ecuador

5 Pediatric Clinic "Dr. Carlos Recalde Cevallos", University of Specialties Espíritu Santo, Samborondón, Ecuador

6 Type C Maternal and Child Health Center, Latin American School of Medicine, Posorja, Ecuador

7 Children's Hospital "Dr. Francisco de Icaza Bustamante", Autonomous Regional University of the Andes, Guayaquil, Ecuador

8 Medical Center Lives Plus, National University of Chimborazo, Ecuador

9 Catholic University of Santiago de Guayaquil, Ecuador

10 InstaSalud, University of Guayaquil, Ecuador

*Address all correspondence to: jahidalgoacosta@hotmail.com; dracalderonleon@hotmail.es; natalyy280@hotmail.com; psolorzano@uees.edu.ec; mariuxi.viteri91@gmail.com; spaul1502@hotmail.com; briggitte_carol1996@hotmail.com; wenbelen04@gmail.com; cirugiacapilar@drpelo.org and anthonymerinoe97@hotmail.com

References

[1] Hidalgo Acosta J, Cobeña Vera J, Guzñay Muñoz D, Rivera Moreira L, Defaz Freire P, Zúñiga Arreaga L, et al. Mortality from sepsis in the intensive care unit. CAMbios-HECAM [Internet]. 2023;**22**(1):E865. Available from: https://revistahcam.iess.gob.ec/index.php/cambios/article/view/865 [Accessed: November 26, 2023]

[2] Robertson KD, Nagra N, Mehta D. Esophageal Candidiasis. Treasure Island (FL): StatPearls Publishing; 2023

[3] Mora Carpio AL, Climaco A. Fungemia Candidiasis. Treasure Island (FL): StatPearls Publishing; 2023

[4] Phongkhun K, Pothikamjorn T, Srisurapanont K, Manothummetha K, Sanguankeo A, Thongkam A, et al. Prevalence of ocular candidiasis and *Candida endophthalmitis* in patients with candidemia: A systematic review and meta-analysis. Clinical Infectious Diseases. 2023;**76**(10):1738-1749. DOI: 10.1093/cid/CIAD064

[5] Xu Z, Huang T, Min D, Soteyome T, Lan H, Hong W, et al. Regulatory network controls microbial biofilm development, with *Candida albicans* as a representative: From adhesion to dispersal. Bioengineered. 2022;**13**(1):253-267. DOI: 10.1080/21655979.2021.1996747

[6] Okoye CA, Nweze E, Ibe C. Invasive candidiasis in Africa, what is the current outlook? Pathogens and Disease. 2022;**80**(1):FTAC012. DOI: 10.1093/femspd/ftac012

[7] Wang B, Wang Y, Zhang L, Lu F, Zhang M, Xu Y. Surveillance study of epidemiology, antifungal susceptibility and risk factors of invasive candidiasis in critically ill patients. Clinical Laboratory. 1 Jun 2022;**68**(6):1257-1264. DOI: 10.7754/Clin.Lab.2021.211001

[8] McCarty TP, White CM, Pappas PG. Candidemia and invasive candidiasis. Infectious Disease Clinics of North America. 2021;**35**(2):389-413. DOI: 10.1016/j.idc.2021.03.007

[9] Ferrando G, Castagnola E. Prophylaxis of invasive fungal infection in neonates: A narrative review for practical purposes. Journal of Fungi (Basel). 2023;**9**(2):164. DOI: 10.3390/jof9020164

[10] Thomas-Rüddel DO, Schlattmann P, Pletz M, Kurzai O, Bloos F. Risk factors for invasive Candida infection in critically ill patients: A systematic review and meta-analysis. Chest. 2022;**161**(2):345-355. DOI: 10.1016/j.chest.2021.08.081

[11] De Kort EA, Buil JB, Schalekamp S, Schaefer-Prokop C, Verweij PE, Schaap NPM, et al. Invasive fungal disease in patients with myeloid malignancies: A retrospective cohort study of a diagnostic-driven care pathway withholding mould-active prophylaxis. Journal of Fungi (Basel). 2022;**8**(9):925. DOI: 10.3390/jof8090925

[12] Franco D, Quindos Andrés G, De La Fuente I, Ribacoba L, Fernández Rodríguez M, Guridi A, et al. Comparative study of invasive candidiasis in Mexico and Spain. In: Proceedings of MOL2NET'17, Conference on Molecular, Biomed., Comput. & Network Science and Engineering. 3rd ed. Basel, Switzerland: MDPI; 2017. DOI: 10.3390/mol2net-03-04596

[13] Peng Z, Tang J. Intestinal infection of *Candida albicans*: Preventing the

formation of biofilm by *C. Albicans* and protecting the intestinal epithelial barrier. Frontiers in Microbiology. 2022;**12**:783010. DOI: 10.3389/fmicb.2021.783010

[14] Kuruoğlu T, Çelik M, Çelmeli F, Tanyel E. *Candida albicans* CARD9 mutation in a patient with meningoencephalitis; a case report [CARD9 mutation in a patient with *Candida albicans* meningoencephalitis; a case report]. Microbiology Bulletin. 2021;**55**(4):656-664. Turkish. DOI: 10.5578/MB.20219717

[15] Scurek M, Pokojova E, Doubkova M, Brat K. Allergic bronchopulmonary candidiasis: A review of the literature and a case report. BMC Pulmonary Medicine. 2022;**22**(1):132. DOI: 10.1186/s12890-022-01921-3

[16] Diba K, Makhdoomi K, Nasri E, Vaezi A, Javidnia J, Gharabagh DJ, et al. Emerging Candida species isolated from renal transplant recipients: Species distribution and susceptibility profiles. Microbial Pathogenesis. 2018;**125**:240-245. DOI: 10.1016/j.micpath.2018.09.026

[17] Jawale CV, Biswas PS. Local antifungal immunity in the kidney in disseminated candidiasis. Current Opinion in Microbiology. 2021;**62**:1-7. DOI: 10.1016/j.mib.2021.04.005

[18] Barantsevich N, Barantsevich E. Diagnosis and treatment of invasive candidiasis. Antibiotics (Basel). 2022;**11**(6):718. DOI: 10.3390/antibiotics11060718

[19] Mellinghoff SC, Hoenigl M, Koehler P, Kumar A, Lagrou K, Lass-Flörl C, et al. EQUAL Candida score: An ECMM score derived from current guidelines to measure QUAlity of clinical Candidaemia management. Mycoses. 2018;**61**(5):326-330. DOI: 10.1111/myc.12746

[20] Vázquez-Olvera R, Volkow P, Velázquez-Acosta C, Cornejo-Juárez P. Candida bloodstream infection in patients with cancer: A retrospective analysis of an 11-year period. Revista Iberoamericana de Micología. 2023;**40**(1):3-9. DOI: 10.1016/j.riam.2022.12.002

[21] Chatelon J, Cortegiani A, Hammad E, Cassir N, Leone M. Choosing the right antifungal agent in ICU patients. Advances in Therapy. 2019;**36**(12):3308-3320. DOI: 10.1007/s12325-019-01115-0

[22] Pristov KE, Ghannoum MA. Resistance of Candida to azoles and echinocandins worldwide. Clinical Microbiology and Infection. 2019;**25**(7):792-798. DOI: 10.1016/j.cmi.2019.03.028

[23] Szekely J, Rakchang W, Rattanaphan P, Kositpantawong N. Fluconazole and echinocandin resistance of Candida species in invasive candidiasis at a university hospital during pre-COVID-19 and the COVID-19 outbreak. Epidemiology and Infection. 2023;**151**:e146. DOI: 10.1017/S0950268823001346

[24] Roilides E, Carlesse F, Tawadrous M, Leister-Tebbe H, Conte U, Raber S, et al. Safety, efficacy and pharmacokinetics of anidulafungin in patients 1 month to <2 years of age with invasive candidiasis, including Candidemia. The Pediatric Infectious Disease Journal. 2020;**39**(4):305-309. DOI: 10.1097/INF.0000000000002568

[25] Tang BHE, Bay JW, Yeong FM, Samuel M. Efficacy and safety of echinocandin monotherapy and combination therapy for immunocompromised patients with systemic candidiasis: A systematic

review and meta-analysis. Journal of Medical Mycology. 2023;**33**(2):101362. DOI: 10.1016/j.mycmed.2023.101362

[26] Auriti C, Falcone M, Ronchetti MP, Goffredo BM, Cairoli S, Crisafulli R, et al. High-dose Micafungin for preterm neonates and infants with invasive and central nervous system candidiasis. Antimicrobial Agents and Chemotherapy. 2016;**60**(12):7333-7339. DOI: 10.1128/AAC.01172-16

[27] Hidalgo Acosta JA, Pozo Gómez CA, Quiñonez Avilez JE, Arteaga Muñoz JL, López Alcívar GN, Sanga Pintag DA, et al. Acute interstitial pneumonia due to pulmonary mycosis. Clinical case presentation. Mediciencias UTA [Internet]. 2023;**7**(2):47-52. Available from: https://revistas.uta.edu.ec/erevista/index.php/medi/article/view/1980 [Accessed: December 12, 2023]

[28] Thompson GR 3rd, Soriano A, Cornely OA, Kullberg BJ, Kollef M, Vazquez J, et al. Rezafungin versus caspofungin for treatment of candidaemia and invasive candidiasis (ReSTORE): A multicentre, double-blind, double-dummy, randomised phase 3 trial. Lancet. 2023;**401**(10370):49-59. DOI: 10.1016/S0140-6736(22)02324-8

[29] Roilides E, Carlesse F, Leister-Tebbe H, Conte U, Yan JL, Liu P, et al. A prospective, open-label study to assess the safety, tolerability and efficacy of anidulafungin in the treatment of invasive candidiasis in children 2 to <18 years of age. The Pediatric Infectious Disease Journal. 2019;**38**(3):275-279. DOI: 10.1097/INF.0000000000002237

[30] Kim J, Nakwa FL, Araujo Motta F, Liu H, Dorr MB, Anderson LJ, et al. A randomized, double-blind trial investigating the efficacy of caspofungin versus amphotericin B deoxycholate in the treatment of invasive candidiasis in neonates and infants younger than 3 months of age. The Journal of Antimicrobial Chemotherapy. 2020;**75**(1):215-220. DOI: 10.1093/jac/dkz398

[31] Kullberg BJ, Viscoli C, Pappas PG, Vazquez J, Ostrosky-Zeichner L, Rotstein C, et al. Isavuconazole versus caspofungin in the treatment of candidemia and other invasive Candida infections: The ACTIVE assay. Clinical Infectious Diseases. 2019;**68**(12):1981-1989. DOI: 10.1093/CID/CIY827

[32] Spec A, Pullman J, Thompson GR, Powderly WG, Tobin EH, Vazquez J, et al. MSG-10: A phase 2 study of oral ibrexafungerp (SCY-078) after initial echinocandin-therapy in non-neutropenic patients with invasive candidiasis. Journal of Antimicrobial Chemotherapy. 2019;**74**(10):3056-3062. DOI: 10.1093/JAC/DKZ277

[33] Pappas PG, Vazquez JA, Oren I, Rahav G, Aoun M, Bulpa P, et al. Clinical safety and efficacy of novel antifungal, fosmanogepix, for the treatment of candidaemia: Results from a phase 2 trial. The Journal of Antimicrobial Chemotherapy. 2023;**78**(10):2471-2480. DOI: 10.1093/jac/dkad256

Chapter 4

Environmental and Social Determinants Related to Candidiasis

Karen del Carmen Morales-Ramírez, Raúl Avila-Sosa, Teresa Soledad Cid-Pérez, Fabiola Avelino-Flores, Esperanza Duarte-Escalante and Ricardo Munguía-Pérez

Abstract

Environmental, social, and economic factors are decisive for susceptibility to infectious diseases caused by opportunistic pathogens, such as *Candida*. Their incidence has increased significantly in recent years, mainly due to a greater number of immunocompromised people, the social and economic environment in which they develop and the current environmental crisis, climate change, which exacerbates health inequalities. Therefore, a literature review was conducted on the main social and environmental determinants of health and virulence factors as determinants of *Candida* spp. infection. Several studies provide valuable insights into the main predisposing determinants of *Candida* colonization and infection in relation to the health status of people and the virulence factors of the aetiological pathogen itself. Although there are some studies on the prevalence of *Candida* in different social classes, there are still few criteria to derive or claim an objective opinion on the social conditions under which this opportunistic pathogen occurs. Therefore, an overall picture that takes into account not only the intrinsic factors of the individual (human biology, health status, etc.) but also the social determinants of health, which may be related to differences in colonization and infection by different *Candida* species, is still lacking.

Keywords: candidiasis, *Candida*, predisposing factors, socioeconomic factors, social determinants of health

1. Introduction

Lifestyle, human biology, health care, and natural and socioeconomic environment are factors that determine a person health status and are collectively referred to as social determinants of health (SDH) [1]. Different circumstances, in which people are born and develop, are crucial for the emergence and spread of emerging diseases as a result of environmental changes [2], lifestyle, human biology, and the distribution of economic resources [1, 3, 4]. Emerging diseases caused by emerging pathogens include opportunistic fungal infections, which are a major cause of morbidity and mortality and are responsible for approximately 1.5 million deaths per year worldwide [5]. The fourth most common cause of all nosocomial fungal infections associated with increased risk factors is mainly due to *Candida* species [6].

Candidiasis is a disease caused by various species of the genus *Candida*. These are yeast fungi that are part of the human microbiome and can be the most common opportunistic fungal pathogens in various infections of the skin, mucous membranes, deep structures, and internal organs [7]. *Candida albicans* is the main cause of nosocomial infections in the bloodstream, known as candidemia [8]. Factors responsible for variations in the prevalence of *Candid*a include the clinical setting, nutritional factors, geographic location, pharmacological therapies, invasive devices, immunosuppressive and chronic degenerative diseases, and hygienic conditions [9–13]. Due to the above factors, the emergence of non-albicans *Candida* species as opportunistic pathogens has been observed in recent years, particularly in underdeveloped countries, especially in vulnerable patients [11]. There is evidence that their emergence is due to the probably indiscriminate use of prophylactic and therapeutic antifungal agents [14], with a clear tendency toward more resistance [15, 16]; on the other hand, adaptation to climate change has had a strong impact on the pathogenicity of fungi. *Candida* spp. can also form biofilms and possess other virulence factors that protect them from the action of various antifungal agents. The aim of this literature review is, therefore, to outline the determinants that favor the development of *Candida* spp. with social determinants being of particular interest, and to examine the influence that the environment, particularly climate change, has on the pathogenicity of emerging species.

2. *Candida* and candidiasis, an overview

Candida belongs to Kingdom: Fungi, Phylum: Ascomycota, Subphylum: Ascomycotina, Class: Ascomycetes, Order: Saccharomycetales, Family: Saccharomycetaceae, and Genus: *Candida*. It is a dimorphic yeast that exhibits different morphological forms under different environmental conditions. For example, *C. albicans* and *C. dubliniensis* can form germ tubes and thick-walled chlamydoconidia in addition to yeast-like cells, whereas *C. glabrata* only has yeast-like cells. *Candida* yeasts are about 2–6 X 3–9 μm in size, depending on the species [7, 17, 18]. *C. albicans* use glucose as a carbon source and amino acids as nitrogen sources [19]. The cell wall of *Candida* spp. consists of mannan (20%), β-(1,3)-d-glucan (50 to 70%), chitin (10 to 20%), proteins (3 to 6%), lipids (1 to 5%), and pigments (melanin). Electron microscopic studies show differences in the organization and composition of the cell wall in the two different morphogenetic forms of this yeast [20]. The cell wall is important for the control of cell permeability and protection against osmotic and mechanical stress. It mediates interaction with the environment *via* adhesins and a large number of receptors that, when activated, trigger a complex signaling cascade within the cell [21]. Ergosterol is the most abundant sterol and is characteristic of the cell membrane. It provides stability, rigidity, and resistance to physical stress factors [21, 22].

Many species of the genus *Candida* are part of the normal biota of the skin, mucous membranes, and gastrointestinal tract of animals and humans; others have been isolated from soil, food, and hospital environments. Between 30 and 70% of healthy people carry at least one *Candida* species [23]. This genus comprises about 200 identified species, 20 of which have caused candidiasis. Ten species (*C. albicans,*

C. glabrata, C. parapsilosis, C. tropicalis, C. guilliermondii, C. famata, C. kefyr, C. krusei, C. lusitaniae and *C. dubliniensis*) are most frequently associated with the various clinical forms of this mycosis [7] and can affect both healthy and immunocompromised patients. An important finding is the identification of the species *Candida auris*, which has emerged as a global public health threat in recent years. *C. auris* poses a major challenge in hospitals as it is difficult to detect, resistance to multiple drugs, changes in its virulence factors, has a high patient mortality rate in patients, and is able to survive on surfaces for long periods of time [6, 24].

Candida is a common inhabitant of the skin and mucous membranes and is part of the natural microbiota of the human body. When its nature changes or the host organism's resistance to *Candida* decreases, it can multiply excessively and cause local, disseminated, or systemic infections of the skin, mucous membranes, deeper structures, and internal organs, which is known as candidiasis [2]. The severity of the infection depends mainly on the primary alterations of the host and less on the pathogenic properties of the fungus. Most infections are endogenous, that is, they are caused by yeasts that are part of the patient's indigenous microbiota [25]. However, infection can also originate from exogenous sources, such as intravenous catheters or cardiac prostheses, especially when these are used in immunodeficient patients [20]. There are also reports of Candida infections in immunocompetent patients without corresponding signs or symptoms [26]. The most common forms of candidiasis are those with superficial involvement, including vulvovaginitis and skin and nail infections [27].

Predisposing factors for candidiasis include extreme age (childhood or old age), increased concentrations of sex hormones such as estrogen in pregnancy (increased vaginal glycogen) creating a carbon-rich environment [28], occlusion of epithelial surfaces (by dentures or occlusive dressings), immune dysfunction (secondary: E.g. HIV/AIDS, leukemia, corticosteroid therapy), chemotherapy (immunosuppressants, antibiotics), endocrine diseases (diabetes mellitus), carcinomas, damaged nail folds, and others [29]. The fourth most common cause of all nosocomial infections associated with increased risk factors is mainly due to *Candida* species [6].

According to various epidemiological studies, about 90% of infections caused by *Candida* are due to five species, including *C. albicans*, and non-albicans such as *C. tropicalis, C. parapsilosis, C. glabrata,* and *C. krusei* [14, 30]. However, *C. albicans* is still the main culprit for invasive infections [18, 31, 32]. Today, the list of reported species continues to grow as molecular diagnostics are used to identify them at the species level, which, given the differences in virulence and drug sensitivity, helps to optimize the treatment of infections caused by species other than *C. albicans* [33, 34].

3. Superficial candidiasis

In superficial mycoses, fungi colonize the outermost keratinized layers of the skin, hair, and nails [35]. They are associated with changes in the hydration and pH of the skin, mouth, throat, and other superficial tissues [7]. Superficial candidiasis is divided into cutaneous and mucocutaneous. The former can manifest as intertrigo in folds, diaper dermatitis, paronychia, and candida onychomycosis, which can be acute or chronic. Superficial candidiasis is one of the most common clinical forms and is typically chronic and recurrent; it can also be the onset of systemic infection [29]. Mucocutaneous candidiasis includes oral candidiasis, digestive tract candidiasis (which can be superficial if invasion is limited to the mucosa and submucosa) [36], vaginitis, balanitis, bronchial, and pulmonary candidiasis. Chronic mucocutaneous candidiasis and *Candida* granuloma are forms of disseminated and deep candidiasis [20].

4. Systemic candidiasis

Over 90% of deaths from mycoses or invasive fungal infections (IFI) are due to candidiasis, aspergillosis, cryptococcosis, and pneumocystosis. Invasive candidiasis, the most widespread of these, leads to severe illness and death, especially in critically ill patients and people with weakened immune systems [15, 16]. With the increasing number of invasive medical procedures and the growing number of immunocompromised patients, an increased incidence of invasive candidiasis caused by non-albicans *Candida* species, including *C. auris*, a yeast with potential for nosocomial transmission that has spread rapidly worldwide, has been observed [37, 38].

Primary risk factors for IFI include neutropenia with less than 500 neutrophils/ml lasting longer than 10 days, blood-related cancers, bone marrow transplants, prolonged corticosteroid treatment of more than 4 weeks, long-term ICU stays of more than 7 days, chemotherapy, HIV infection, invasive medical procedures, and recently administered immunosuppressive drugs. Other risk factors include malnutrition, solid organ transplants, severe burns, major surgery, patients receiving parenteral nutrition, and the use of intravascular catheters [26].

Invasive candidiasis, which is often associated with hospitalization, involves blood infections (candidemia) and serious infections such as intra-abdominal abscesses, peritonitis and osteomyelitis [39], pneumonia [40], ocular candidiasis [26], endocarditis [41], candiduria [42], and fungal infection in the central nervous system [43]. Almost all organs can become secondarily infected after hematogenous dissemination of the fungus [19].

5. Virulence factors and resistance

Virulence factors allow *Candida* spp. to rapidly adapt to different host niches and cause infections in patients with risk factors. The strategies used to combat the host's natural defense mechanisms are strongly influenced by the environment [38]. Virulence factors include: (a) the expression of surface molecules to achieve attachment of the microorganism to host cells using adhesion proteins; (b) the formation of biofilms is clinically important as their spatial arrangement facilitates the penetration of nutrients, and excretion of waste products [44], they are more resistant to antifungal drugs and provide protection from host's immune defenses [45, 46]; therefore, *Candida* spp. can colonize long-term medical devices, such as intravascular catheters, and the cells can separate and lead to widespread infection [38, 47]; (c) secretion of hydrolytic enzymes that promote penetration and destruction of surrounding tissue, thereby releasing nutrients from host cells [48] and toxins such as candidalysin, a cytolytic peptide toxin that is essential for systemic and mucosal infections and enables epithelial damage [49]; (d) the ability to change its morphology (dimorphism), characterized by the morphological transition from blastoconidia to hyphae, and the form of transition between these are pseudohyphae [35]; (e) tigmotropism, a mechanism that allows invasion of invaginations [48]; (f) its metabolic adaptability due to a phenotypic change and response to stress mediated by heat shock proteins (HSP) [38, 50].

Several studies have shown that, unlike other *Candida* species, *C. auris* has adapted to hostile environments as it can grow at high temperatures (> 40°C) and tolerates high salt concentrations (> 10% NaCl, wt/vol) [51].

5.1 Resistance

Years of use of antifungal and antibacterial substances in agriculture and healthcare have altered the global microbiome, leading to an increase in fungal infections that are resistant to drugs in plants, animals, and humans [37, 52].

The sensitivity to antifungal agents can differ among various *Candida* species and even among strains of the same species. Resistance to microbes can develop with any type of antifungal agents, making the treatment of candidemia more complex [30]. While resistance to multiple drugs is uncommon, there is a growing number of reports on inherent and developed resistance to several drugs (azoles, echinocandins, and polyenes) in various *Candida* species, particularly in *C. glabrata* and more recently in *C. auris*. In general, non-albicans species are associated with increased resistance and high mortality rates [53, 54]. First-line drugs, including echinocandins and azoles, have been effective, but resistance has increased in *Candida* species due to indiscriminate prophylactic and therapeutic use [52, 55]. Other factors responsible for increased resistance include subtherapeutic drug concentrations at infection/colonization sites, sequestration of the drug in the biofilm matrix [56], overexpression of the drug target (e.g. efflux pumps), development of compensatory pathways for ergosterol production, and activation of cellular stress responses [57, 58]. Recent research suggests that mutations of DNA repair genes for mating defects may facilitate the acquisition of resistance genes, which has been observed in *C. glabrata* [53].

Studies, in the USA, have reported a low incidence of fluconazole resistance in *C. albicans*, approximately 0.5 to 2%. In contrast, higher rates of resistance have been reported in *C. tropicalis, C. parapsilosis,* and *C. glabrata:* 4 to 9%, 2 to 6%, and 11 to 13%, respectively. The emerging yeast *C. auris* can have a resistance rate up to 93% to fluconazole, 35% to amphotericin B, and 7% to echinocandins [58]. On the other hand, several studies have observed that strains of *C. glabrata* exhibited reduced susceptibility to one or more echinocandins in addition to resistance to fluconazole [57, 59].

6. Environmental determinants conducive to the development of candidiasis

6.1 Adaptability to different environmental conditions and climate change

Clinically important *Candida* species have been isolated from different environmental sources whose substrates could be their main reservoirs or environmental niches. Therefore, it is important and necessary to conduct more studies that consider the ecological triad: Pathogen-Host-Environment. Environmental conditions, such as global warming and climate change, are a favorable scenario for the change and adaptability of different microorganisms.

There are several papers of great importance reporting the presence of *C. auris* in clinical settings and its potential to spread rapidly among patients. Arora et al. [59] found *C. auris* in samples of beach sand and wetlands in the Andaman Islands, India. Casadevall et al. [60] hypothesized that *C. auris* acts as an environmental fungus that may have existed as a saprophytic plant in specialized ecosystems, such as wetlands.

The emergence of *C. auris* could be due to the rise in global temperatures due to anthropogenic climate change, which led to the selection of thermotolerant strains and their combined tolerance to salinity, resulting in its emergence as a pathogenic fungus in humans that has a wide geographic range. According to Casadevall et al. [61], the discovery of *C. auris* at two locations on the remote Andaman Islands confirms its status as an environmental organism, a necessary prerequisite for the hypothesis.

On the other hand, *C. albicans* is not only a commensal yeast of humans and animals but also has been detected in soils, freshwater, seawater, vegetables, and wetlands [62]. Studies by Nunn et al. [63] showed the presence of *C. dubliniensis* in ticks associated with seabirds in Ireland. *C. tropicalis* has been detected in agricultural fields, forest soils, oil, and mud contaminated soils, fresh and seawater, beach sand, rivers and lakes, sugar cane bagasse, and coconut water [64]. *C. parapsilosis*, a ubiquitous microorganism, is part of the human microbiota and colonizes mucous membranes, skin, and nails. *C. auris* is widely distributed in nature and is often found in various nonhuman sources such as domestic animals, insects, soil, seawater, and plants [65, 66]. *C. glabrat*a is a species commonly found in the environment, especially from various sources such as water, soil, surfaces, and plants [67]. In another study, the presence of *C. glabrata* was detected in the gut microbiota of yellow-legged gulls [68]. Randhawa et al. [69] isolated *C. kruse*i from the decaying wood of *Ficus religios*a, and it has also been isolated from mammals, birds, springs, and fruits [70]. Another unusual *Candid*a species that rarely infects humans is *C. melibiosica*, which is often isolated from rivers and oceans, but there are also studies reporting its presence in some traditional beers. However, in 2010, the first case of nosocomial fungemia in an 82-year-old patient caused by *C. melibiosica* was described [71].

Global warming and climate change have a significant impact on the pathogenicity and survival of fungi, as well as on the environmental reservoir of the pathogen. Adaptation to higher temperatures increases its ability to multiply in the human body, which has a high basal temperature. This leads to an increased potential for disease, even in species previously considered nonpathogenic. This affects the spread of fungi as the increase in heat-resistant species facilitates interaction with humans, infection and transmission through skin contact, inhalation, and/or ingestion [2, 72].

7. Contamination of the clinical environment and the hands of healthcare personnel

One of the risk factors for invasive fungal infection (IFI) in immunocompromised patients is prolonged hospitalization. IFIs with *Candida* spp. associated with hospitalizations are associated with 20 to 40% of all deaths, with a mortality rate of 15 to 35% in adults and 10 to 15% in newborns. Nearly 50% of candidemia episodes occur in intensive care units, contributing to prolonged hospitalization and significant healthcare costs [14, 34], with mortality ranging from 40 to 60% [33, 73, 74].

In healthcare settings, contaminated surfaces in the environment contribute significantly to the spread of infectious diseases. Despite regular cleaning, some microorganisms can form biofilms that lead to permanent contamination. In addition to reducing susceptibility to antimicrobials and biocides, biofilms also protect microorganisms from a hostile environment, including desiccation over extended periods of time [75].

In a study by Welsh et al. [76], the ability of *C. auris* and *C. parapsilosis* to persist on common plastic surfaces in healthcare settings was investigated. The results showed that *C. auris* remained viable for at least 14 days and *C. parapsilosis* for at least 28 days. In addition, Kramer et al. [77] reported that *C. albicans* survived on surfaces for up to 4 months. In another study, persistence of various *Candida* species in the hospital environment was reported on both dry and mostly moist surfaces, indicating a potential route of spread for emerging multidrug-resistant fungal pathogens, such as *C. auris* [78] and colonization or infection of hospital patients and healthcare workers [75].

Although most *Candida* infections originate from endogenous sources, it is increasingly reported that the hands of healthcare workers serve as carriers for pathogen transmission. Sakita et al. [79] investigated the susceptibility of five yeasts (*C. albicans, C. parapsilosis, C. glabrata, C. tropicalis,* and *C. krusei*) isolated from the hands of healthcare workers (physicians, nurses, and assistants) to different antifungal agents. Their results showed that the hand isolates had high resistance rates, with *C. glabrata* being the most resistant and *C. parapsilosis* the most common. In another study conducted in a neonatal intensive care unit in Brazil, *Candida* species were isolated from the hands of healthcare workers, including isolates of *Candida* spp., *C. parapsilosis sensu stricto, C. parapsilosis sensu, C. metapsilosis, C. orthopsilosis, C. famata, C. albicans, C. lusitaniae, C. kefyr, C. krusei, C. glabrata, C. tropicalis,* and *C. guilliermondii* [80]. Delfino, Scordino [81], reported the presence of yeasts on the hands of nurses, orderlies, residents, and physicians in three intensive care units of a hospital in Milan, Italy. Approximately, 39% of the healthcare staff tested positive for yeast. *C. parapsilosis* was the most frequently isolated species followed by *C. albicans, C. glabrata, C. tropicalis, C. lambica, C. lusitaniae,* and *C. krusei*.

A study conducted by Kordecka et al. [82] in a hospital in Poland revealed a high prevalence of *Candida*, with *C. albicans*, *C. glabrata*, and *C. krusei* being the predominant species in samples collected from cell phones and especially on the hands of medical staff. Community data show that the frequency of colonization of the hands of hospital staff with yeasts of the genus *Candida* is about 20% for medical staff and 80% for nursing staff and paramedical assistants. This shows how environmental factors, such as the hospital environment, directly influence the colonization of individuals with the genus *Candida* [83, 84].

7.1 HIV/aids

Both acquired and congenital immunodeficiencies can be associated with an increased susceptibility to systemic infections [26]. Immunocompromised patients have an increased risk of candidemia and deep infections with visceral disease [33].

HIV/AIDS is the most common factor associated with oropharyngeal candidiasis in children and adolescents. It is directly related to low peripheral blood CD4+ T lymphocyte counts, below 200 cells/μL, so its presence has been used as a clinical marker for infection, prior antifungal use, and changes in the oral environment [85]. In contrast to oropharyngeal candidiasis, it has been observed that patients with HIV/AIDS who develop esophageal candidiasis have lower CD4+ T lymphocyte counts [86]. The presence of oropharyngeal or esophageal candidiasis is considered an indicator of inmunosuppression [87].

C. dubliniensis has a high prevalence in the oral cavities of people infected with the human immunodeficiency virus [57], and other associated species in both HIV-infected children and adults are *C. albicans* and *C. glabrata* [85]. In a study conducted in Kerman, Iran, to compare the demographic characteristics and frequency of *Candida* species causing oropharyngeal infection between patients with HIV/AIDS and individuals without HIV, it was found that both groups differed significantly in terms of species prevalence. According to the results, *C. albicans* was the most common species isolated from patients with HIV/AIDS, followed by *C. glabrata*, and other species isolated were included *C. parapsilosis, C. krusei,* and *C. kefyr* [87].

7.2 Nutritional factors

The root causes of child malnutrition include lack of access to food, lack of health care, use of unsafe water and sanitation systems, and poor care and feeding practices. These underlying problems are caused by conflict, inadequate education, poverty, gender inequality, inadequate infrastructure, and other fundamental problems [88]. Globally, malnutrition is the leading of immunodeficiency and is considered a risk factor for infant death. Malnutrition has been found to increase the risk of oral colonization with *Candida* by 4.5 to 5.3 times compared to apparently healthy infants. In this study, the *Candida* species found in children aged 6 to 13 years with malnutrition were *C. albicans, C. tropicalis, C. krusei,* and *C. glabrata* [10]. Lu [89] reported a high prevalence of oral *Candida* spp. infections in patients (males and females aged 16 to 76 years) from a hospital in Kaohsiung, Taiwan, who had iron deficiency anemia. A high incidence of oral *Candida* infections was found in 85% of patients with iron deficiency. Another study reported that malnourished infants and low birth weight infants were at increased risk of *C. parapsilosis* infection due to the administration of parenteral nutrition to ICU patients [90]. In a study of 18 of 54 patients (older adults) in two geriatric hospitals who had oral candidiasis, it was associated with protein-calorie malnutrition, in addition to other conditions, most notably poor dental hygiene [91]. Another study in France, conducted in hospitalized older adults, found a positive correlation between oral condition, dysphagia, and malnutrition with *Candida* spp. infections [92].

7.3 Chronic degenerative diseases

In the last decade, the increase in the immunocompromised population has led to a high incidence of invasive *Candida* infections [93]. Diabetes mellitus (DM) is one of the most common endocrine diseases, affecting the immune system. Patients with DM are susceptible to opportunistic infections due to elevated serum glucose levels and a weakened cellular immune system [94]. Type 2 diabetes mellitus (DM2), which affects ninety percent of people, is primarily associated with personal lifestyle, including a high-calorie diet, lack of physical activity, and smoking [93]. Several studies have shown that patients with DM are more likely to be oral *Candida* carriers and have an increased risk of candidiasis, which is related to poor metabolic control, neutrophil dysfunction, decreased salivary flow, increased blood and salivary glucose concentrations, and poor immune response. It is well known that patients with diabetes mellitus are more susceptible to fungal infections, especially *C. albicans* [95, 96]. In a study by Aitken et al. [95] in Chile, five *Candida* species were identified, with *C. albicans* being the most common followed by *C. glabrata, C. tropicalis* and *C. guilliermondii* in saliva samples from people with DM2.

In Shiraz, Iran, Zomorodian et al. [94] conducted a study on the prevalence of oral *Candida* colonization in patients with DM1 and DM2. The results showed different *Candida* species of the oral mucosa, with *C. albicans* being the predominant species, followed by *C. dubliniensis, C. glabrata, C. parapsilosis, C. guilliermondii, C. krusei, C. kefyr*, and *C. tropicalis*. One population at potential risk for candidemia is patients with cancer. Both hematologic and solid neoplasms have been reported to be predictors of this infection. In addition, this infection could worsen the prognosis of malignant diseases (30-day mortality is up to 56%). According to the results of a study on the epidemiology and risk factors of candidemia in cancer patients in a cancer center in China, mortality was significantly higher than that of bacterial bloodstream infections, with *C. albicans* being the leading pathogen, followed by *C. parapsilosis, C. tropicalis, C. glabrata, C. lusitaniae*, and *C. famata*. In addition to hematologic and solid neoplasms, total parenteral nutrition, urinary catheters, cancer metastases in distant organs, and gastrointestinal cancers were shown to be predictors of candidemia [97].

Clinical data on candidemia in adult cancer patients reported that *C. albicans* was the most common species in both hematologic and oncologic patients. In hematologic patients, *C. albicans* was the most common species, followed by *C. parapsilosis, C. krusei,* and *C. glabrata*, while in oncologic patients, the second most common species was *C. glabrata,* followed by *C. parapsilosis* and only one case of candidemia due to *C. krusei* in an oncologic patient. Other isolated species were *C. tropicalis, C. guilliermondii, C. kefyr, C. lusitanae, C. famata, C. rugosa,* and *C. sake* [98].

The increased susceptibility of cancer patients to *Candida* infections is largely due to the weakening of innate immune cells and epithelial barriers caused by chemotherapy. These are the body's main defense mechanisms against fungal infections. In addition, conventional chemotherapeutic agents have a negative effect on the components of the adaptive immune system that play a crucial role in the antifungal response [99].

7.4 Extreme age

According to the literature, the prevalence of oral candidiasis in newborns varies between 4 and 15%, with *C. albicans* most commonly associated with thrush. The prevalence of invasive candidiasis correlates with low birth weight [100] and prolonged hospitalization, affecting 2 to 20% of newborns. It accounts for 10% of all cases of sepsis in low birth weight neonates (<1500 g) and is the second most common cause of death due to opportunistic infections [101]. Several surveillance studies have shown that most cases of invasive candidiasis in infants and neonates are due to *C. parapsilosis* as a first or second cause, both in Europe and North America [90]. In particular, CNS candidiasis in neonates is largely due to the immaturity of the physical (blood-brain) barrier to *Candida* spp. [102].

*Candid*a colonization increases with age because older adults have several metabolic disorders, including decreased liver and kidney function, use of multiple medications, and malnutrition. As the immune system deteriorates with age, this leads to increased susceptibility to infectious diseases, reduced response to vaccines, higher incidence of cancer, and an increase in autoimmune and other chronic diseases. Both the innate and adaptive immune responses are impaired by the aging process [103]. Studies based on oral cavity cultures in middle-aged and older adults have identified *C. albicans, C. glabrata, C. parapsilosis*, and *C. tropicalis* [104]. It has been observed that *C. glabrata* in particular is more common in adults than in children and neonates [57]. In the geriatric population, oral candidiasis is one of the three main reasons for consultation due to stomatitis caused by the use of dentures [105].

7.5 Hygienic conditions

Candida grows on surfaces and often colonizes dentures, leading to denture stomatitis or subplate stomatitis. The diagnosis of denture stomatitis is important. According to Ibañez et al. [105], about 50% of the people in their study population with an average age of 65 to 74 years and 70% from 75 to 84 years used removable dentures. Regarding the factors associated with the development of subplaque candidiasis, in the studies conducted in different populations, the colonization of the surface of removable dentures by *Candida* species is mainly attributed to the poor or absent hygiene that patients perform both in the oral cavity and on their dentures.

Another condition that is particularly common in young children and the elderly who live in poor hygienic conditions is intertrigo caused by *Candida*, which is favored by the following factors: Moisture, heat, friction, and maceration [106].

7.6 Occupational exposure

There are different types of occupational hazards that can cause various clinical manifestations, most of which are superficial and cause high morbidity in the working population. A link has been observed between working conditions and dermatological diseases. An example of this is intertrigo and onychomycosis of the hands, which is not only related to the humid environment but also to contact with highly sugary foods processed by bakers, cooks, manual strawberry pickers, fruit packers, food handlers, or food shippers, in which case it is an occupational disease [20]. Leal et al. [107] investigated superficial mycoses in 21 workers of a metal smelting company, 81% of whom were infected [17] with some type of dermatomycosis. Five cases belonged to intertriginous candidiasis caused by *C. albicans*. The authors concluded that the high incidence of superficial mycosis (including candidiasis) among the workers was due to the environmental conditions in the workplace such as humidity, high temperature, personal hygiene in a communal bathroom, and occlusive footwear for long working hours.

Silias et al. [108] carried out a study on 109 female workers (seamstresses) in a lingerie factory in Puebla, Mexico, 56 of whom had athlete's foot. The laboratory data showed that *Candida* spp. grew in 15 patients, with women being the most affected, as well as patients with diabetes mellitus, carriers of systemic lupus erythematosus, and the only patient with leukemia. The authors conclude that the following factors predispose to the development of an athlete's foot: the heat generated by the machines, the duration of exposure, the wrapping of the foot by synthetic footwear, and poor personal hygiene. Occupational mycoses can seriously harm the working population.

8. Epidemiology

The epidemiology of candidemia and the distribution of *Candid*a species varies over time, between geographic regions and hospitals, and under the considerable influence of patient characteristics, antifungal drug administration, and clinical practices [109]. Although *C. albicans* is considered the most common and virulent cause of candidemia worldwide, currently, more than half of candidemia cases are attributed to non-albicans *Candid*a species, mainly *C. parapsilosis, C. glabrata, C. krusei, a*nd *C. tropicalis*, as well as other emerging pathogens such as *C. auris*, probably as a consequence of the increasing use of azoles, echinocandins or other prophylactic/therapeutic antifungals [14, 32]. This is consistent with the 20-year surveillance study of the SENTRY antifungal surveillance program 1997–2016, which observed that the overall proportion of infections attributable to *C. albicans* decreased from 57.4 to 46.4% [110]. In the USA, more than 30% of candidemia cases are now caused by *C. glabrata*, with other commonly isolated species being *C. tropicalis* and *C. parapsilosis* a worrying trend given the higher rates of antifungal resistance in associated with this species [37, 111]. In northwestern Europe, as in the USA, the second most common species is generally *C. glabrata*. In Latin America, southern Europe, India, and Pakistan, *C. parapsilosis* and *C. tropicalis* are found more frequently than *C. glabrata* [111].

Determinants	Main effects	References
Virulence factors	Surface molecules Biofilm Secretion of hydrolytic enzymes and toxins Dimorphism Metabolic adaptability Tigmotropism	[35, 44–50, 116]
Antifungal resistance	Intrinsic and acquired resistance Indiscriminate use of antifungals (Varies according to each *Candid*a species and even within strains of the same species)	[30, 53–58]
Adaptation to different environmental conditions	Beach sand, wetlands, soils (agricultural, forestry, contaminated with oil and mud), fresh water, seawater, rivers, springs, decomposing plants and vegetables, domestic and wild animals, insects	[59–71]
Adaptation to climate change / global warming	Acclimatization to higher temperatures enhances human interaction	[2, 60, 61, 72]
Contamination of different environments	Clinical environment (hospitalization)	[75–78]
	Healthcare personnel's hands	[79–82]
HIV/AIDS	Oropharyngeal Candidiasis	[57, 85, 87, 117]
	Esophageal candidiasis	[86]
	Candidemia	[26, 33]
Nutrition	Malnutrition	[10, 90–92]
	Iron deficiency anemia	[89]
Chronic degenerative diseases	DM1	[94]
	DM2	[94, 95]
	Hematologic and solid neoplasms	[97, 98]
Age extremes	Newborns (immature immune system)	[90, 100, 102]
	Older adults (immune system weakened by aging)	[57, 103–105]
Hygiene	Lack of hygiene (stomatitis and intertrigo)	[105, 118]
Occupational exposure	Superficial candidiasis (Intertrigo, onychomycosis)	[20, 107, 108]

Table 1.
Main determinants associated with candidiasis.

The rapid emergence and spread resistant *C. auris* [39] have significantly altered the epidemiology of candidemia in different geographical locations and healthcare facilities as it has become a major cause of invasive infections [112]. As of February 2021, *C. auris* has been reported in 47 countries [113]. The first isolate was reported in late May 2020 from the bloodstream of a patient with severe endometriosis and multiple gastrointestinal complications; the infection subsequently spread to 12 patients in the ICU [114, 115].

Table 1 shows a summary of the main determinants of *Candid*a colonization infection, which include intrinsic factors of the etiological agent (virulence factors, resistance to fungi, adaptation to different environments and climate change) and risk factors related to the host (immunosuppression, habits, occupation, and hospitalization).

9. Social determinants of health in the context *Candid*a infection

9.1 Social determinants of health (SDH)

The World Health Organization (WHO) defines health as a state of complete physical, mental, and social well-being and not merely the absence of disease. This definition makes it possible to consider different perspectives such as the social aspects of health as social determinants of health [119].

SDH are the social, economic, and environmental conditions that influence an individual's state of health. According to the World Health Organization (WHO), SDH such as education, housing, nutrition, work environment, access to services, unemployment, and health care are essential for equitable health. In recent years, it has also become widely accepted that the socioeconomic conditions in which people live strongly influence their chances of good health. Health and illness follow a social gradient: The lower a person's socioeconomic position, the lower their chances of good health [120].

Poor environmental, social, and economic conditions have a negative impact on health, increase susceptibility to infectious diseases caused by emerging pathogens; these factors contribute to health inequalities that can span multiple generations. Technological advances, increasing unplanned urbanization, and climate change are new and emerging trends that may exacerbate existing inequalities and further increase inequalities in health opportunities and outcomes [121].

9.2 State of the art in DSS associated with candidiasis

One of the populations that are particularly vulnerable to opportunistic infections is those living in poverty, who suffer from precarious health conditions and have limited or no access to health facilities [122]. For example, dermatophytosis is more common in people living in crowded or promiscuous conditions such as in barracks, prisons, or nursing homes, where confined spaces favor contact with infectious material. Subcutaneous mycoses, such as mycetoma, sporotrichosis, and chromoblastomycosis, are common in underdeveloped countries, due to the fact that agricultural activities are performed manually, while in highly developed countries, they do not occur and the cases observed are imported [123]. Therefore, below are several some articles describing some social factors that favor the development of *Candida* spp. The available published research articles on socioeconomic factors were retrieved and reviewed from three reliable databases: PubMed, Google Scholar, and Scopus, with a total of 31 articles. The search was performed using the keywords: "*Candida*," "candidiasis," and "socioeconomic," in both English and Spanish and without limiting the date of publication as there is little information on this topic. The selection of articles was based on the title, abstract, and in some cases, related documents.

Of the publications found describing sociodemographic characteristics or socioeconomic factors of patients colonized or infected with *Candida*, 29 articles referred to superficial infections and/or colonization, of which the most common clinical form was vulvovaginal with 20 (65%) publications followed by oral colonization and/or candidiasis (7; 23%) and 2 (6%) onychomycoses. Only 2 (6%) published articles on systemic candidiasis or candidemia were found (**Table 2**). The prevalence of *Candid*a colonization/infection was estimated based on the total number of patients with *Candid*a and the total population.

Regarding vulvovaginal candidiasis, only 12 out of 20 studies showed any kind of positive association between socioeconomic factors and clinical manifestations. In addition, **Table 1** lists these factors or determinants observed in the different populations studied. López Martínez et al. [124] conducted a study of 600 obstetric-gynecology patients to investigate opportunistic factors in vaginal candidiasis. In relation to the total population and the number of patients with a positive test for *Candida*, the prevalence was 43.5% (261), of which 134 (22.3%) had this yeast as a part of the microbiota and in 127 (21.2%) it was considered a pathogen more frequently observed in patients of middle socioeconomic level. It was also found that pregnancy, followed by an association between pregnancy, malnutrition, and anemia, were the most common opportunistic factors for the development of vaginal candidiasis. *C. albican*s was the most common species (67.7%) followed by *C. tropicali*s (18.8%), *C. stellatoide*a (8.7%), *C. pseudotropicalis* (2.4%), *C. parakrusei* (1.6%), and C. guillermondi (0.8%). Studies by Spinillo et al. [125], in an obstetrics and gynecology clinic at the University of Pavia, Italy, found that patients with vaginal infections caused by *C. glabrat*a compared to *C. albican*s had lower educational and socioeconomic levels, were associated with recurrent vaginal candidiasis, and were more common in women over 38 years of age. The prevalence of *Candida* infection was 33.1% (786/2374) in the population, with *C. albicans* being the most common species (79.5%) followed by *C. glabrata* (10.9%) and to a lesser extent other species such as *C. tropicalis, C. kefyr,* and *C. parapsilosi*s.

In another study conducted in Paraguay by Laspina et al. [126] between 1995 and 1996 in 196 girls with a clinical diagnosis of vulvovaginitis, it was that the prevalence of this infection caused by *Candida* spp. was 21.5%. The characteristics of the population studied showed that the girls generally came from families with a medium to low socioeconomic level, 50% of the mothers had secondary education, and 44.4% had only primary education. Lassey et al. [127] determined the transmission rates of potential lower genital tract pathogens and factors associated with colonization in 200 women with incomplete abortion treated at a hospital in Accra, Ghana. As a result, they found a combination of bacterial vaginosis and *C. albicans* in 17.2% (34 patients) of the study population and a significant association with the presence of potential pathogens and people living in an urban slum, malnutrition, and anemia, factors characteristic of low socioeconomic status.

In a population-based study of women in Goa, India, Patel et al. [128] investigated the burden and determinants of reproductive tract infections in 2432 patients. The results showed a population-wide prevalence of *Candida* of 8.5% (206 cases). Analysis of socioeconomic risk factors for candidiasis showed that this infection was

Clinical manifestation	Year	Geographic region	Characteristics of the population	Related species	Prevalence (%)	DSS	References
Vulvovaginal Candidiasis (CVV)	1984		600 obstetrics-gynecology outpatients	*C. albicans, C. tropicalis, C. stellatoidea, C. kefyr, C. parapsilosis, C. guilliermondi*	43.5% (261)	Pregnancy, malnutrition, anemia, *medium socioeconomic status	[124]
	1995	Pavia, Italia	2374 gynecological patients from a vaginitis cliniC	*C. albicans, C. glabrata, C. tropicalis, C. kefyr y C. parapsilosis.*	33.1% (786)	*Women older than 38 years, lower educational and socioeconomic levels in patients with *C. glabrata*.	[125]
	2005	Paraguay	196 pediatric gynecological patients	*Candida sp.*	—	*Lower-middle socioeconomic level, primary and secondary parental education	[126]
	2004	Accra, Ghana	200 patients undergoing manual vacuum aspiration	*C. albicans*	17.2% [34]	Housing in marginal urban neighborhood	[127]
	2006	Goa, India	2432 gynecological patients	*Candida sp.*	8.5% (206)	Younger age, not being of Muslim origin, fewer children in the household, not having tap water in the house	[128]
	2018	Odisha, India	558 non-pregnant gynecological patients of reproductive age	*C. albicans*	34% (190)	Lack of hygiene, lower educational level	[129]
	2014	China	1341 gynecological patients	*Candida spp.*	51.37% (689)	Low educational level, older age, marriage, vaginal douching	[130]
	2022	19 countries worldwide	Pregnant patients	*C. albicans, C. glabrata, C. krusei, C. tropicalis, C. lypolytica, C. kefyr, C. famata, C. parapsilosis y C. dubliniensis*	17–90%	Age, gestational age, parity, low educational, and socioeconomic levels	[131]
	2020	Latin America	Gynecological patients of reproductive age	*C. albicans*	20–50%	Early sexual life, socioeconomic inequality, use of contraceptive methods, multiple partners, unprotected sexual activity	[132]

DOI: http://dx.doi.org/10.5772/intechopen.1004600

Clinical manifestation	Year	Geographic region	Characteristics of the population	Related species	Prevalence (%)	DSS	References
	2012	Detroit, MI, U.S.A.	25 patients referred to a Vaginitis Clinic	*C. albicans*	100%	*Married and insured white women with more than 12 years of formal education, average or above average socioeconomic level.	[133]
	2013	Juiz de Fora, Brazil	69 gynecological patients with CVV	*C. albicans, C. glabrata, C. lusitaniae*	100%	*White women, higher education, and married.	[134]
	1995	Taipei, Taiwán	17,047 gynecological patients	*Candida spp.*	3.4% (580)	College education or higher, age in adolescence.	[135]
Colonization and/or oral candidiasis	2014	Bolivia	75 elderly patients	*C. albicans*	61.3% [46]	Physiological changes, low defenses, poor hygiene, malnutrition, low income, low education.	[136]
	2012	México	60 children with HIV/AIDS 60 malnourished children 57 Tarahumara children	*C. albicans, C. tropicalis* *C. albicans, C. krusei, C. tropicalis, C. glabrata* *C. albicans, C. krusei*	57.1% [36] 38.2% [27] 17.5% [11]	Immunosuppression Immunosuppression, * underlying causes —	[122]
	2011	São Paulo, Brasil	117 pediatric AIDS patients	*C. albicans, C. tropicalis, C. kefyr, C. krusei, C. glabrata, C. guilliermondii*	62% [86]	Low socioeconomic level	[137]
	2022	U.S.A.	101 infants	*C. albicans, C. krusei, C. glabrata*	48% [48]	Presence of *S. mutans*, maternal factors: oral carriage of *C. albicans*, lower education, disadvantaged socioeconomic status, more than three decayed teeth.	[138]
	2001	Piracicab, SP, Brasil	239 children	*C. albicans, C. tropicalis, C. krusei, C. parapsilosis*	47.3% [113]	—	[139]
	2019	U.S.A.	48 pregnant patients	*C. albicans, C. krusei, C. glabrata, C. tropicalis, C. dubliniensis*	100%	Socioeconomic disadvantage, hypertension, number of decayed teeth, level of *S. mutans* in saliva.	[140]
	2012	U.S.A.	249,092 patients diagnosed with oral candidiasis	*Candida spp.*	100%	Residence in geographic areas of low socioeconomic strata, comorbid condition	[141]

Clinical manifestation	Year	Geographic region	Characteristics of the population	Related species	Prevalence (%)	DSS	References
Nail, cutaneous and mucosal candidiasis	2006	México	3749 patients from rural communities	*C. parapsilosis, C. albicans, C. guilliermondii, C. tropicalis, C. humicola, C. famata*	0.58% [22]	Marginalization	[142]
	2006	Manaos, Brasil	394 with clinical suspicion of superficial mycosis	*Candida spp., C. albicans*	18.3% [72]	Middle social class	[143]
Candidemia	2020	Grecia	522,197 hospitalized patients	*C. albicans, C. parapsilosis* complex, *C. glabrata complex, C. tropicalis, C. krusei, Candida spp.*	0.082% (429)	Economic crisis (limited resources for medical care), solid organ malignancies	[74]
	2016	U.S.A.	225 patients with home parenteral nutrition	*Candida spp.*	6.22% [14]	Anticoagulant therapy, ulcers or open wounds, public health insurance (low socioeconomic status)	[144]

**Predominance of factors in the population, but not a statistically significant relationship.*

Table 2.
Social determinants of health in Candida *infection-colonization.*

significantly associated with younger age, non-Muslim origin, fewer children in the household, and lack of tap water in the home. The latter could have an impact on poor personal hygiene and social inequality, as factors Torondel et al. [129] found in a hospital in Odisha, India, to determine whether poor hygiene practices during menstruation were associated with three common lower reproductive tract infections. The data showed that *C. albicans* infection was the second most common (34%; 190) among the three types of infections. Women with this disease rarely practiced personal hygiene. In addition, socioeconomic studies showed that the prevalence of candidiasis was inversely proportional to a higher level of education.

In 2013, Na et al. [130] conducted a study in two tropical regions of China (Hainan and Sanya) in which they investigated the risk factors associated with genital tract infection caused by *Candida* spp. in 689 infected gynecological patients. The prevalence of Candida was 51.37% (689/1341). Age, low education, marriage, and vaginal douching were significant risk factors for *Candida* infection. Patients with higher levels of education were unlikely to be infected with *Candida* species and the incidence increased with age, which differs from the situation described by Wang et al. [135], where candidiasis decreased with age. Disha et al. [131] conducted a review study in which they investigated the prevalence and risk factors for vulvovaginal candidiasis (VVC) in pregnant women worldwide. The data collected indicate a high prevalence of CVV in pregnant women worldwide, particularly in Asian and African countries, with Kenya, Nigeria, and Yemen having rates of 90.38%, 62.2%, and 61.5%, respectively. However, the prevalence of CVV in pregnant women worldwide ranged from the lowest 17% (Selangor, Malaysia) to the highest 90% (Kenya). They also found that the prevalence of CVV during pregnancy varied with age (25–29 years), gestational period (last trimester), parity (multiple births), and low educational and socioeconomic level. The differences in prevalence rates worldwide may be due to geographical, ethnic, and socioeconomic factors, as well as differences in sampling and culture techniques.

In 2022, Duran Cañarte et al. [132] investigated the most common risk factors for vaginal infections in women of childbearing age in Latin America. The results showed that the main pathogens associated with vaginal infections in women aged 15 to 40 years were *Gardnerella vaginalis, Trichomonas vaginalis,* and *C. albicans*. In addition, the study found that *C. albicans* was the most common pathogen in countries such as Argentina 2018 (25%), Colombia 2018 (20.3%), Ecuador 2018 (50%), Peru 2019 (22.3%), Cuba 2019 (20–25%), and Mexico 2017 (20%). It was concluded that the most predisposing risk factors for acquiring vaginal infections include early sexual life, socioeconomic inequality, the use of contraceptive methods, multiple partners, and unprotected sexual activity. In contrast, a study by Marchaim et al. [133], conducted between 2000 and 2010, examined the incidence of vulvovaginitis due to fluconazole-resistant *C. albicans* and risk factors in female patients at a hospital in Detroit, MI. They found 25 cases of women with recurrent vaginitis over an 11-year period. Most patients were primarily married insured white women with more than 12 years of formal education and average or above average socioeconomic status.

Tavares Rodrigues et al. [134] conducted a study to investigate the epidemiologic profile of patients with vulvovaginal candidiasis (VVC) in Juiz de Fora, Brazil. Of the patients studied, aged 15 to 52 years, 79.7% were white women, 58% had higher education, 56.5% were married, and 97.1% were sexually active. The study showed that the most prevalent species were *C. albicans* (98.1%), followed by *C. glabrata* (5.4%) and only 3 with C. *lusitaniae*. Although sociodemographic characteristics such as age, marital status, and education were not significantly related to vulvovaginal candidiasis, this study showed a predominance of the disease in participants who were considered white, college educated, and married.

Wang et al. [135] investigated the epidemiological differences between candidiasis and trichomonads in cytological smears from 17,047 patients attending health centers and clinics in Taipei, Taiwan. The overall prevalence of *Candida* infection was 3.4%. Infection was higher in adolescents and decreased with age, especially in over 60 years of age. Adolescence showed a positive correlation with candidiasis as an independent risk factor, with indices of socioeconomic status and education (higher education or higher compared to illiterate women). There was no clear association between ethnicity and hygiene and candidiasis. On the other hand, eight publications were found in which sociodemographic factors of patients with vulvovaginal candidiasis such as socioeconomic and educational level, age, place of residence, occupation, behavior/habits, marital status, health services, and ethnicity were investigated or described, but no associations were found or were present as determinants for the development of candidiasis [145–152].

Regarding socioeconomic factors in oral *Candida* infection/colonization, effects have been reported in the elderly, pregnant women, especially in the pediatric population. A study by Atalaya et al. [136] examined the prevalence of oral candidiasis in 75 elderly patients attending a medical consultation in a hospital in Bolivia. Candida was observed in 61.3% [46] of the study population. The predominant factors for the prevalence of oral candidiasis include physiological changes, age-related low defenses, poor oral hygiene habits, poor eating habits, low income, and low education, which favor infection with *C. albicans*. Gaitán Cepeda et al. [122] investigated the presence of *Candid*a in the oral cavity of children susceptible to opportunistic infections and whether there is an association between this oral colonization and three types of at-risk populations. The results in the HIV/AIDS (n = 60) and malnutrition (n = 60) groups showed the highest frequency of *Candida* (51.7% and 38.2%, respectively), with the highest frequency of *C. albicans* isolates followed by *C. tropicalis* in HIV/AIDS patients; the malnutrition group showed the highest diversity, where *C. albicans* was most common, followed by *C. krusei* and only one isolate of *C. tropicalis, C. glabrata* and *Candida* spp. In the third group, Tarahumara children (n = 57), one of the poorest ethnic populations in Mexico, the frequency was similar to the control group (n = 29) (17.5% and. 10.3% respectively), with the most frequent species being *C. albicans* with eight isolates, two of *C. krusei* and one *Candida s*pp. Isolate.

Domaneschi et al. [137] investigated the prevalence of factors associated with oral colonization by *Candida* spp. in pediatric AIDS patients in São Paulo, Brazil. The prevalence of oral *Candida* colonization was 62% (86/117). Only seven children had a clinical manifestation of oral candidiasis. Of the 86 yeast isolates, *C. albican*s was the most prevalent (69 of 86), followed by *C. tropicalis* (5 of 86), *C. kefyr* (4 of 86), *C. krusei* (3 of 86), *C. glabrata* (2 of 86), and *C. guilliermondi*i (1 of 86). In the study, a positive correlation was observed between *Candid*a colonization and sociodemographic characteristics in children. A higher incidence was found in children who did not live in their own home and in children with more than two siblings. These results indicate that people in unfavorable socioeconomic circumstances are more susceptible to *Candida* infections.

In 2022, Alkhars et al. [138] examined *Candida* colonization in the oral cavity of 101 young children from low income and racial minorities in the USA. The results showed that *Candida* colonization and carriage in infants was positively associated with maternal factors such as oral carriage of *C. albicans*, low education, socioeconomic disadvantage, and more than three decayed teeth. In addition, 48% of infants were found to have *Candida* colonization at 6 months of age, which remained at the same level until 12 months of age. The most frequently detected species included *C. albicans* and *C. krusei* followed by *C. glabrata*. In contrast, Moreira et al. [139] studied *Candida* colonization in 239 Brazilian children divided into five different socioeconomic categories (A to E), with D and E being the least favored. The results showed the presence of *Candida* spp. in 47.3% of the samples. *C. albicans* was the most frequently isolated species in all socioeconomic categories, followed by *C. krusei, C. tropicalis,* and *C. parapsilosis*. Furthermore, the prevalence of *Candida* did not differ significantly between the groups. However, a significant correlation was found between caries rates and socioeconomic categories. Nevertheless, it is important to note that recent studies have associated the presence of *Candid*a spp. with a higher prevalence of caries [153].

In a study conducted in the USA by Xiao et al. [140] on oral health and *Candida* colonization in socioeconomically disadvantaged pregnant women, it was found that 24 out of 48 patients had positive *Candid*a detection; moreover, a higher frequency of *Candida* colonization in women was positively associated with hypertension. *C. glabrata, C. krusei, C. tropicalis,* and *C. dubliniensis* were also detected in the study participants. This suggests that more than 10% of socioeconomically disadvantaged pregnant women received only emergency dental treatment to relieve orofacial pain, inflammation, and advanced infections instead of routine prenatal oral health care. The oral health of these patients represents a major health inequality. In addition, Elangovan et al. [141] reported on 249,092 patient visits to the emergency department with a diagnosis of oral candidiasis. The following was found: the percentage of women (55%) with oral candidiasis was slightly higher than the percentage of men; a significantly higher proportion of young people under 19 years of age (32.2%), and many people living in geographical areas with low socioeconomic strata (64%). In addition, nearly all ED visits were found to be associated with ≥1 comorbid condition predisposing to or related to oral candidiasis such as fluid disorders, HIV infection, esophageal disease, nutritional deficiencies, and secondary malignant neoplasms.

In relation to the different dermatophytoses caused either by *Candida* or by other dermatophytes, it is believed that occupation and socioeconomic status are determining factors for these manifestations since patients with low socioeconomic status have a greater physiological impact due to the work they perform (laborers, farmers, artisans, among others) [154]. Méndez Tovar et al. [142] reported in 3749 cases from five Mexican rural communities with a high degree of marginalization that aimed to perform medical consultations with specialists in dermatology and mycology. The overall percentage of dermatoses caused by fungi was high at 13.75% (498); however, only 98 fungi were identified in three municipalities. The study showed that the inhabitants of these municipalities had a high morbidity associated with fungi. A total of 22 isolates (0.58%) belonged to *Candida* causing nail, skin, and mucosal candidiasis, with *C. parapsilosis* being the most frequent, followed by *C. albicans,* and others such as *C. guilliermondii, C. tropicalis, C. humicola, C. famata, Pichia ohmeri,* and *Candida* spp. Probably, the difficult living conditions in which these patients live lead to little attention being paid to these infections. Other pathologies indicative of underdevelopment, such as scabies, acarosis, pediculosis, and malnutrition of varying degrees, were found with great frequency.

De Oliveira et al. [143] examined 394 patients with clinically suspected superficial mycosis, 256 of whom were positive. They concluded that onychomycosis and pityriasis versicolor are the most common mycoses in the Amazon region and that *Candida* spp. (72; 31.57%) and *Malassezia* spp. (77; 33.77%) are the most common pathogens. The prevalence of *Candida* was 18.3%. Superficial mycoses were present in all social classes, but cases were more frequent in people of social class C (97; 37.89%), which is classified as moderate according to the Brazilian classification system.

Siopi et al. [74] reported on a 10-year (2009–2018) retrospective surveillance study in a tertiary hospital in Greece that collected information on the epidemiology of candidemia, especially during severe socioeconomic events (financial crisis). The number of hospitalized patients was 522,197, among whom a total of 429 candidemia attacks were recorded. *C. albicans* was the most common species (41%), followed by *C. parapsilosis* (37%), *C. glabrata* (11%), *C. tropicalis* (7%), *C. krusei* (1%), and *Candida* spp. (3%). They found that incidence of candidemia on internal medicine wards and of *C. parapsilosis* infections increased significantly during this period. It was suggested that the current economic crisis affecting the country may have contributed to candidemia. So limited resources for medical care difficulties in diagnosis. The reduction in specialized hospital staff and the increase in the number of patients in public clinics could have a negative impact on basic infection control measures, rather than being associated with critical differences in the characteristics of the population studied.

Durkin et al. [144] conducted a descriptive observational study of 225 patients discharged with home parenteral nutrition from a hospital in St. Louis, Missouri, USA, between 2007 and 2009. Among the catheter-related complications, infections were identified in 68 patients, of which 14 (20%) involved *Candida*. Predictive factors that were more common in patients who developed a catheter-related bloodstream infection included age, ulcers or open wounds, anticoagulation, and public insurance. This could be because publicly insured patients are generally older and/or have a lower socio-economic status, as stipulated by the admission criteria.

10. Conclusions

Several studies have been reported that provide valuable insights into the major predisposing determinants of *Candida* colonization and infections in relation to the health status of the individual and the virulence factors of *Candida* itself. Although there is some work examining the prevalence of *Candida* in different social classes, as well as a sociodemographic description, there are still few criteria to derive or assert an objective opinion on the social conditions in which this opportunistic pathogen occurs. In this sense, it remains only a poorly documented diagnosis of what might be happening. It is still inaccurate to claim that a particular species is prevalent in certain socioeconomic strata.

So, there is still a lack of a global overview that takes into account the social determinant of health in addition to the intrinsic factors of individuals (human biology, health status, etc.) that could be related to variations in colonization and infection by the different *Candida* species. Research is needed to assess the relationship between socioeconomic characteristics of people (social development, marginalization, the environment in which people live and develop, etc.) and variations in colonization and infection by different *Candida* species, applying a methodology and data analysis with tools such as descriptive and predictive mathematical models that allow understanding the impact of DSS on the development of the disease. This is done with the intention of identifying the social parameters that are more influential (in multispecies candidiasis) and can be controlled.

Acknowledgements

Author Morales-Ramírez gratefully acknowledges financial support for his PhD studies from Natl. Council for Science, Technology and Humanities of Mexico (CONAHCYT).

Conflict of interest

The authors declare no conflict of interest.

Author details

Karen del Carmen Morales-Ramírez[1,2], Raúl Avila-Sosa[1,3], Teresa Soledad Cid-Pérez[2], Fabiola Avelino-Flores[1,4], Esperanza Duarte-Escalante[5] and Ricardo Munguía-Pérez[1,2]*

1 Posgrado en Ciencias Ambientales, Instituto de Ciencias, Ciudad Universitaria, Puebla, México

2 Laboratorio de Micología, Centro de Investigación en Ciencias Microbiológicas, Instituto de Ciencias, Ciudad Universitaria, Puebla, México

3 Departamento de Bioquímica-Alimentos, Facultad de Ciencias Químicas, Benemérita Universidad Autónoma de Puebla, Ciudad Universitaria, Puebla, México

4 Laboratorio de Patogenicidad Microbiana, Centro de Investigación en Ciencias Microbiológicas, Instituto de Ciencias, Ciudad Universitaria, Puebla, México

5 Departamento de Microbiología y Parasitología, Facultad de Medicina, Universidad Nacional Autónoma de México, Ciudad de, México

*Address all correspondence to: ricardo.munguia@correo.buap.mx

References

[1] Urbina-Fuentes M. Marco conceptual de los Determinantes Sociales de la Salud en México. Gaceta Conbioética. 2015; **15**(3):6-11

[2] Tiew PY, Mac Aogain M, Ali NABM, Thng KX, Goh K, Lau KJX, et al. The mycobiome in health and disease: Emerging concepts, methodologies and challenges. Mycopathologia. 2020;**185** (2):207-231

[3] Salvucci E. El agotamiento del bioma y sus consecuencias. Acta Biológica Colombiana. 2013;**18**(1):31-42

[4] Galli A, Pagés M, Swieszkowski S. Factores determinantes de la salud. Kervorkian R, Grancelli H, Blanco P, editors. In: Contenidos Transversales. Buenos Aires: SAC; 2017. pp. 1-8

[5] Jallow S, Govender NP. Ibrexafungerp: A first-in-class oral triterpenoid glucan synthase inhibitor. Journal of Fungi. 2021;7(3):163

[6] Du H, Bing J, Hu T, Ennis CL, Nobile CJ, Huang G. *Candida auris*: Epidemiology, biology, antifungal resistance, and virulence. PLOS Pathogens. 2020;**16**(10):e1008921-e

[7] Manzano-Gayosso P. Candidosis. In: Molina-López J, López-Martínez R, Sánchez-Vega R, editors. Microbiología y Parasitología Médicas de Tay. 1.5th ed. Méndez Editores: Mexico; 2019. pp. 892-896

[8] Reyes-Montes MR, Duarte-Escalante E, Martínez-Herrera E, Acosta-Altamirano G, Frías-De León MG. Current status of the etiology of candidiasis in Mexico. Revista Iberoamericana de Micología. 2017; **34**(4):203-210

[9] Lazo V, Hernández G, Méndez R. Candidiasis sistémica en pacientes críticos, factores predictores de riesgo. Horizonte Médico (Lima). 2018;**18**(1): 75-85

[10] Gaitán-Cepda LA, Sánchez-Vargas LO, Pavia-Ruiz N, Muñoz-Hernández R, Villegas-Ham J, Caballos-Salobreña A. Candida bucal en niños mexicanos con VIH/sida, desnutrición o marginación social. Revista Panamericana de Salud Pública. 2012;**31**(1):48-53

[11] Hanna MC. Clinical manifestations of candidiasis: Beyond Candida albicans. Virology & Immunology Journal. 2019;**3**(3):1-22

[12] Méndez-Tovar LJ. Generalidades de las micósis. In: López-Martínez R, editor. Microbiología y Parasitología Médicas de Tay. 1.5th ed. Mexico: Méndez Editores; 2019. pp. 856-558

[13] Pereira LC, Correia AF, da Silva ZDL, de Resende CN, Brandão F, Almeida RM, et al. Vulvovaginal candidiasis and current perspectives: New risk factors and laboratory diagnosis by using MALDI TOF for identifying species in primary infection and recurrence. European Journal of Clinical Microbiology & Infectious Diseases. 2021;**40**(8):1681-1693

[14] Alobaid K, Ahmad S, Asadzadeh M, Mokaddas E, Al-Sweih N, Albenwan K, et al. Epidemiology of Candidemia in Kuwait: A nationwide, population-based study. Journal of Fungi. 2021;7(8):673

[15] Quindós G. Epidemiology of candidaemia and invasive candidiasis. A changing face. Revista Iberoamericana de Micología. 2014;**31**(1):42-48

[16] Quindós G, Marcos-Arias C, San-Millán R, Mateo E, Eraso E. The

continuous changes in the aetiology and epidemiology of invasive candidiasis: From familiar Candida albicans to multiresistant *Candida auris*. International Microbiology. 2018;**21**(3):107-119

[17] Hernández F. Generalidades de los hongos. In: López-Martínez R, editor. Microbiología y Parasitología Médica de Tay. 5th ed. Mexico: Méndez Editores; 2019. pp. 851-855

[18] Hameed AR, Ali SM, Ahmed LT. Biological study of *Candida* species and virulence factor. International Journal of Advanced Research in Engineering & Technology. 2018;**1**(4):8-16

[19] Talapko J, Juzbašić M, Matijević T, Pustijanac E, Bekić S, Kotris I, et al. Candida albicans—The virulence factors and clinical manifestations of infection. Journal of Fungi. 2021;**7**(2):79

[20] Arenas R. Micología Médica. 5th ed. México: Interamericana Editores; 2014. 239-60 p

[21] Gow NAR, Latge J-P, Munro CA. The fungal cell wall: Structure, biosynthesis, and function. Microbiology Spectrum. 2017;**5**(3):1-25

[22] Jordá T, Puig S. Regulation of ergosterol biosynthesis in *Saccharomyces cerevisiae*. Genes. 2020;**11**(7):795

[23] Gow NAR, Yadav B. Microbe profile: Candida albicans: A shape-changing, opportunistic pathogenic fungus of humans. Microbiology. 2017;**163**(8): 1145-1147

[24] Spivak ES, Hanson KE. *Candida auris*: An emerging fungal pathogen. Journal of Clinical Microbiology. 2018; **56**(2):1588-1617

[25] Gigliotti N. Microbiota intestinal: Sus repercusiones clínicas en el cuerpo humano. Archivos Argentinos de Pediatria. 2013;**111**(6):523-527

[26] Badiee P, Hashemizadeh Z. Opportunistic invasive fungal infections: Diagnosis & clinical management. The Indian Journal of Medical Research. 2014;**139**(2):195-204

[27] Land Curi AL, Wanke B, Vasconcelso-Santos DV, Oréfice F. Candidiasis. In: Zierhut M, Pavesio C, Ohno S, Orefice F, Rao NA, editors. Intraocular Inflammation. Berlin, Heidelberg: Springer; 2016. pp. 1261-1267

[28] Pineda-Murillo J, Cortés-Figueroa AA, Uribarren-Berrueta TNJ, Castañón-Olivares LR. Candidosis vaginal. Revisión de la literatura y situación de México y otros países latinoamericanos. Revista Médica Risaralda. 2017;**23**(1):34-38

[29] Hay RJ. Superficial Mycoses. In: Magill A, Ryan ET, Hill D, Solomon T, editors. Hunter's Tropical Medicine and Emerging Infectious Diseases. Beijing: Elsevier; 2020. pp. 610-615

[30] Medeiros MAP, Melo APV, Bento AO, Souza LBFC, Neto FAB, Garcia JB-L, et al. Epidemiology and prognostic factors of nosocomial candidemia in Northeast Brazil: A six-year retrospective study. PLoS One. 2019;**14**(8):e0221033-e

[31] Ng KP, Kuan CS, Kaur H, Na SL, Atiya N, Velayuthan RD. *Candida* species epidemiology 2000–2013: A laboratory-based report. Tropical Medicine & International Health. 2015; **20**(11):1447-1453

[32] Bongomin F, Gago S, Oladele R, Denning D. Global and multi-national prevalence of fungal diseases—Estimate precision. Journal of Fungi. 2017;**3**(4):57

[33] Freeman Weiss Z, Leon A, Koo S. The evolving landscape of fungal diagnostics, current and emerging microbiological approaches. Journal of Fungi. 2021;**7**(2):127

[34] McCarty TP, Pappas PG. Invasive Candidiasis. Infectious Disease Clinics of North America. 2016;**30**(1): 103-124

[35] Murray PR, Rosenthal KS, Pfaller MA. Microbiología Médica. 8th ed. Madrid: Elsevier; 2017. 556-678 p

[36] Stamatiades GA, Ioannou P, Petrikkos G, Tsioutis C. Fungal infections in patients with inflammatory bowel disease: A systematic review. Mycoses. 2018;**61**(6):366-376

[37] Friedman S. Emerging fungal infections: New patients, new patterns, and new pathogens. Journal of Fungi. 2019;**5**(3):67

[38] Ciurea CN, Kosovski I-B, Mare AD, Toma F, Pintea-Simon IA, Man A. Candida and Candidiasis—Opportunism versus pathogenicity: A review of the virulence traits. Microorganisms. 2020; **8**(6):857

[39] Pappas PG, Lionakis MS, Arendrup MC, Ostrosky-Zeichner L, Kullberg BJ. Invasive candidiasis. Nature Reviews Disease Primers. 2018;**4**(1): 18026

[40] Godoy MCB, Ferreira Dalla Pria HR, Truong MT, Shroff GS, Marom EM. Invasive fungal pneumonia in immunocompromised patients. Radiologic Clinics of North America. 2022;**60**(3):497-506

[41] Mamtani SS, Aljanabi NM, Gupta Rauniyar RP, Acharya A, Malik BH. Candida endocarditis: A review of the pathogenesis, morphology, risk factors, and Management of an Emerging and Serious Condition. Cureus. 2020;**12**(1):1-7

[42] Aghili SR, Abastabar M, Soleimani A, Haghani I, Azizi S. High prevalence of asymptomatic nosocomial candiduria due to Candida glabrata among hospitalized patients with heart failure: A matter of some concern? Current Medical Mycology. 2021;**6**(4):1-8

[43] Chaussade H, Cazals X, Desoubeaux G, Jouvion G, Bougnoux M-E, Lefort A, et al. Central nervous system candidiasis beyond neonates: Lessons from a nationwide study. Medical Mycology. 2021;**59**(3):266-277

[44] Wall G, Montelongo-Jauregui D, Vidal Bonifacio B, Lopez-Ribot JL, Uppuluri P. Candida albicans biofilm growth and dispersal: Contributions to pathogenesis. Current Opinion in Microbiology. 2019;**52**:1-6

[45] Silva S, Henriques M, Martins A, Oliveira R, Williams D, Azeredo J. Biofilms of non- *Candida albicans Candida* species: Quantification, structure and matrix composition. Medical Mycology. 2009;**47**(7):681-689

[46] Pereira R, Santos Fontenelle RO, Brito EHS, Morais SM. Biofilm of *Candida albicans*: Formation, regulation and resistance. Journal of Applied Microbiology. 2021;**131**(1):11-22

[47] Ramage G, Rajendran R, Sherry L, Williams C. Fungal biofilm resistance. International Journal of Microbiology. 2012;**2012**:1-14

[48] Polke M, Hube B, Jacobsen ID. Candida survival strategies. Advances in Applied Microbiology. 2015;**91**:139-235

[49] Naglik JR, Gaffen SL, Hube B. Candidalysin: Discovery and function in

Candida albicans infections. Current Opinion in Microbiology. 2019;**52**: 100-109

[50] Soll DR. The role of phenotypic switching in the basic biology and pathogenesis of *Candida albicans*. Journal of Oral Microbiology. 2014;**6**(1): 22993

[51] Wang X, Bing J, Zheng Q, Zhang F, Liu J, Yue H, et al. The first isolate of *Candida auris* in China: Clinical and biological aspects. Emerging Microbes & Infections. 2018;**7**(1):1-9

[52] Fisher MC, Hawkins NJ, Sanglard D, Gurr SJ. Worldwide emergence of resistance to antifungal drugs challenges human health and food security. Science. 2018;**360**(6390):739-742

[53] Arendrup MC, Patterson TF. Multidrug-resistant Candida: Epidemiology, molecular mechanisms, and treatment. The Journal of Infectious Diseases. 2017;**216**(Suppl. 3):S445-SS51

[54] Arastehfar A, Carvalho A, Nguyen MH, Hedayati MT, Netea MG, Perlin DS, et al. COVID-19-associated candidiasis (CAC): An underestimated complication in the absence of immunological predispositions? Journal of Fungi. 2020;**6**(4):211

[55] Lee Y, Puumala E, Robbins N, Cowen LE. Antifungal drug resistance: Molecular mechanisms in *Candida albicans* and beyond. Chemical Reviews. 2021;**121**(6):3390-3411

[56] Mayer FL, Wilson D, Hube B. *Candida albicans* pathogenicity mechanisms. Virulence. 2013;**4**(2):119-128

[57] Pristov KE, Ghannoum MA. Resistance of Candida to azoles and echinocandins worldwide. Clinical Microbiology and Infection. 2019;**25**(7): 792-798

[58] Berkow E, Lockhart S. Fluconazole resistance in *Candida* species: A current perspective. Infection and Drug Resistance. 2017;**10**:237-245

[59] Arora P, Singh P, Wang Y, Yadav A, Pawar K, Singh A, et al. Environmental isolation of *Candida auris* from the coastal wetlands of Andaman Islands, India. MBio. 2021;**12**(2):1-9

[60] Casadevall A, Kontoyiannis DP, Robert V. Environmental *Candida auris* and the global warming emergence hypothesis. MBio. 2021;**12**(2):1-3

[61] Casadevall A, Kontoyiannis DP, Robert V. On the emergence of *Candida auris*: Climate change, azoles, swamps, and birds. MBio. 2019;**10**(4):1397-1419

[62] Sautour M, Lemaître JP, Ranjard L, Truntzer C, Basmaciyan L, Depret G, et al. Detection and survival of *Candida albicans* in soils. Environmental DNA. 2021;**3**(6):1093-1101

[63] Nunn MA, Schäefer SM, Petrou MA, Brown JRM. Environmental source of Candida dubliniensis. Emerging Infectious Diseases. 2007;**13**(5):747-750

[64] Lima R, Ribeiro FC, Colombo AL, de Almeida JN. The emerging threat antifungal-resistant Candida tropicalis in humans, animals, and environment. Frontiers in Fungal Biology. 2022;**3**:3-6

[65] Branco J, Miranda IM, Rodrigues AG. Candida parapsilosis virulence and antifungal resistance mechanisms: A comprehensive review of key determinants. Journal of Fungi. 2023;**9**(1):80

[66] van Asbeck EC, Clemons KV, Stevens DA. Candida parapsilosis: A

review of its epidemiology, pathogenesis, clinical aspects, typing and antimicrobial susceptibility. Critical Reviews in Microbiology. 2009;**35**(4): 283-309

[67] Hassan Y, Chew SY, Than LTL. Candida glabrata: Pathogenicity and resistance mechanisms for adaptation and survival. Journal of Fungi (Basel, Switzerland). 2021;7(8):1-18

[68] Al-Yasiri MH, Normand A-C, L'Ollivier C, Lachaud L, Bourgeois N, Rebaudet S, et al. Opportunistic fungal pathogen Candida glabrata circulates between humans and yellow-legged gulls. Scientific Reports. 2016;**6**:36157

[69] Randhawa HS, Mussa AY, Khan ZU. Decaying wood in tree trunk hollows as a natural substrate for Cryptococcus neoformans and other yeast-like fungi of clinical interest. Mycopathologia. 2001; **151**(2):63-69

[70] Gómez-Gaviria M, Mora-Montes HM. Current aspects in the biology, pathogeny, and treatment of candida krusei, a neglected fungal pathogen. Infection and Drug Resistance. 2020;**13**: 1673-1689

[71] Lim HJ, Lee OJ, Kim SH, Shin MG, Shin JH. First case of nosocomial fungemia caused by candida melibiosica. Annals of Laboratory Medicine. 2020; **40**(2):177-179

[72] Garcia Solache MA, Casadevall A. Global warming will bring new fungal diseases for mammals. mbioasmorg. 2010;**1**(1):1-3

[73] Bassetti M, Righi E, Montravers P, Cornely OA. What has changed in the treatment of invasive candidiasis? A look at the past 10 years and ahead. The Journal of Antimicrobial Chemotherapy. 2018;**73**(Suppl. 1):i14-i25

[74] Siopi M, Tarpatzi A, Kalogeropoulou E, Damianidou S, Vasilakopoulou A, Vourli S, et al. Epidemiological trends of Fungemia in Greece with a focus on Candidemia during the recent financial crisis: A 10-year survey in a tertiary care academic hospital and review of literature. Antimicrobial Agents and Chemotherapy. 2020;**64**(3):1516-1519

[75] Ku TSN, Walraven CJ, Lee SA. *Candida auris*: Disinfectants and implications for infection control. Frontiers in Microbiology. 2018;**9**:1-8

[76] Welsh RM, Bentz ML, Shams A, Houston H, Lyons A, Rose LJ, et al. Survival, persistence, and isolation of the emerging multidrug-resistant pathogenic yeast *Candida auris* on a plastic health care surface. Journal of Clinical Microbiology. 2017;**55**(10): 2996-3005

[77] Kramer A, Schwebke I, Kampf G. How long do nosocomial pathogens persist on inanimate surfaces? A systematic review. BMC Infectious Diseases. 2006;**6**:130

[78] Piedrahita CT, Cadnum JL, Jencson AL, Shaikh AA, Ghannoum MA, Donskey CJ. Environmental surfaces in healthcare facilities are a potential source for transmission of *Candida auris* and other Candida species. Infection Control and Hospital Epidemiology. 2017;**38**(9): 1107-1109

[79] Sakita KM, Faria DR, Silva EM, Tobaldini-Valério FK, Kioshima ES, Svidzinski TIE, et al. Healthcare workers' hands as a vehicle for the transmission of virulent strains of Candida spp.: A virulence factor approach. Microbial Pathogenesis. 2017;**113**:225-232

[80] de Paula MR, Silva FF, Melo SGO, Alves PGV, Brito MO, de Souza

Bessa MA, et al. Characterization of *Candida* species isolated from the hands of the healthcare workers in the neonatal intensive care unit. Medical Mycology. 2018;**57**(5):588-594

[81] Delfino D, Scordino F, Pernice I, Lo Passo C, Galbo R, David A, et al. Potential association of specific Candida parapsilosis genotypes, bloodstream infections and colonization of health workers' hands. Clinical Microbiology and Infection: the Official Publication of the European Society of Clinical Microbiology and Infectious Diseases. 2014;**20**(11):O946-O951

[82] Kordecka A, Krajewska-Kułak E, Łukaszuk C, Kraszyńska B, Kułak W. Isolation frequency of Candida present on the surfaces of mobile phones and handsx. BMC Infectious Diseases. 2016;**16**:238

[83] Strausbaugh LJ, Sewell DL, Ward TT, Pfaller MA, Heitzman T, Tjoelker R. High frequency of yeast carriage on hands of hospital personnel. Journal of Clinical Microbiology. 1994; **32**(9):2299-2300

[84] Zurita MS. Situación de la resistencia antifúngica de especies del género Candida en Perú. Revista Peruana de Medicina Experimental y Salud Pública. 2018;**35**(1):126

[85] Castillo-Martínez NA, Mouriño-Pérez RR, Cornejo-Bravo JM, Gaitán-Cepeda LA. Factores relacionados a candidiasis oral en niños y adolescentes con VIH, caracterización de especies y susceptibilidad antifúngica. Revista Chilena de Infectología. 2018;**35**(4): 377-385

[86] Hoversten P, Otaki F, Katzka DA. Course of Esophageal candidiasis and outcomes of patients at a single Center. Clinical Gastroenterology and Hepatology. 2019;**17**(1):200-2.e1

[87] Hosain Pour A, Salari S, Almani GN, P. Oropharyngeal candidiasis in HIV/ AIDS patients and non-HIV subjects in the southeast of Iran. Current Medical Mycology. 2018;**4**(4):1-6

[88] Sablah M. Causes and Impacts of Undernutrition over the Life Course. New York: UNICEF; 2019

[89] Lu S-Y. Perception of iron deficiency from oral mucosa alterations that show a high prevalence of Candida infection. Journal of the Formosan Medical Association = Taiwan yi zhi. 2016;**115**(8): 619-627

[90] Tóth R, Nosek J, Mora-Montes HM, Gabaldon T, Bliss JM, Nosanchuk JD, et al. Candida parapsilosis: From genes to the bedside. Clinical Microbiology Reviews. 2019;**32**(2):111-118

[91] Tosello A, Chevaux JM, Montal S, Foti B. Assessment of oral status and oro-pharyngeal candidosis in elderly in short-term hospital care. Odonto-stomatologie tropicale = Tropical Dental Journal. 2008;**31**(121):43-48

[92] Poisson P, Laffond T, Campos S, Dupuis V, Bourdel-Marchasson I. Relationships between oral health, dysphagia and undernutrition in hospitalised elderly patients. Gerodontology. 2016;**33**(2):161-168

[93] Nouraei H, Jahromi MG, Jahromi LR, Zomorodian K, Pakshir K. Potential pathogenicity of *Candida* species isolated from oral cavity of patients with diabetes mellitus. BioMed Research International. 2021;**2021**: 9982744

[94] Zomorodian K, Kavoosi F, Pishdad GR, Mehriar P, Ebrahimi H, Bandegani A, et al. Prevalence of oral Candida colonization in patients with

diabetes mellitus. Journal de Mycologie Medicale. 2016;**26**(2):103-110

[95] Aitken-Saavedra J, Lund RG, González J, Huenchunao R, Perez-Vallespir I, Morales-Bozo I, et al. Diversity, frequency and antifungal resistance of *Candida* species in patients with type 2 diabetes mellitus. Acta Odontologica Scandinavica. 2018;**76**(8): 580-586

[96] Lamichhane RS, Boaz K, Natarajan S, Shrestha M. Assessment of Candidal carriage in patients with type II diabetes mellitus. Journal of Pathology of Nepal. 2015;**5**(9):733-738

[97] Li D, Xia R, Zhang Q, Bai C, Li Z, Zhang P. Evaluation of candidemia in epidemiology and risk factors among cancer patients in a cancer center of China: An 8-year case-control study. BMC Infectious Diseases. 2017; **17**(1):536

[98] Slavin MA, Sorrell TC, Marriott D, Thursky KA, Nguyen Q, Ellis DH, et al. Candidaemia in adult cancer patients: Risks for fluconazole-resistant isolates and death. The Journal of Antimicrobial Chemotherapy. 2010;**65**(5):1042-1051

[99] Teoh F, Pavelka N. How chemotherapy increases the risk of systemic candidiasis in cancer patients: Current paradigm and future directions. Pathogens. 2016;**5**(1):6

[100] Weimer KED, Smith PB, Puia-Dumitrescu M, Aleem S. Invasive fungal infections in neonates: A review. Pediatric Research. 2022;**91**(2):404-412

[101] Tinoco-Araujo JE, Araújo DFG, Barbosa PG, Santos PSS, Medeiros AMC. Invasive Candidiasis and Oral Manifestations in Premature Newborns. Einstein (Sao Paulo, Brazil). 2013;**11**(1):71-75

[102] Vigezzi C, Riera FO, Rodriguez E, Icely PA, Miró MS, Figueredo CM, et al. Candidiasis invasora: Un enfoque a la infección en el sistema nervioso central. Revista Argentina de Microbiología. 2021;**53**(2):171-178

[103] Nishimaki F, Yamada S-i, Kawamoto M, Sakurai A, Hayashi K, Kurita H. Relationship between the quantity of Oral Candida and Systemic condition/diseases of the host: Oral Candida increases with advancing age and Anemia. Mycopathologia. 2019; **184**(2):251-260

[104] Baumgardner DJ. Oral fungal microbiota: To thrush and beyond. Journal of Patient-Centered Research and Reviews. 2019;**6**(4):252-261

[105] Ibañez-Mancera NG, Robles-Bonilla C, Lecona-Ayala J. Frecuencia de candidiasis oral asociada al uso de prótesis dentales en pacientes de la Clínica Odontológica de la Universidad Anáhuac Norte. Revista ADM. 2017; **74**(2):74-78

[106] Kaushik N, Pujalte GGA, Reese ST. Superficial fungal infections. Primary Care: Clinics in Office Practice. 2015; **42**(4):501-516

[107] Leal B, González M, Gómez F, Aular L. Micosis superficiales en trabajadores de una empresa de fundición de metales. Dermatología Venezolana. 2006;**44**(3):18-20

[108] Silias-Márquez BE, Enríquez-Guerra MA, Alvarado-González J, Sánchez-Hernández JA, Muñoz-Zurita G, Rivera-Tapía JA. Diagnóstico de laboratorio de candidosis podal en costureros de una fábrica en la ciudad de Puebla. Anales Médicos. 2008;**55**(1):22-27

[109] de Medeiros MAP, de Melo APV, de Oliveira BA, de Souza LBFC, de Assis

Bezerra Neto F, Garcia JBL, et al. Epidemiology and prognostic factors of nosocomial candidemia in Northeast Brazil: A six-year retrospective study. PLoS One. 2019;**14**(8):1-15

[110] Pfaller MA, Diekema DJ, Turnidge JD, Castanheira M, Jones RN. Twenty years of the SENTRY antifungal surveillance program: Results for Candida species from 1997–2016. Open forum. Infectious Diseases. 2019;**6** (Suppl. 1):S79-S94

[111] Lamoth F, Lockhart SR, Berkow EL, Calandra T. Changes in the epidemiological landscape of invasive candidiasis. Journal of Antimicrobial Chemotherapy. 2018;**73**(Suppl. 1): i4-i13

[112] Ahmad S, Alfouzan W. *Candida auris*: Epidemiology, diagnosis, pathogenesis, antifungal susceptibility, and Infection control measures to combat the spread of infections in healthcare facilities. Microorganisms. 2021;**9**(4):807

[113] CDC. *Candida auris*. Atlanta: Centers for Disease Control and Prevention; 2021

[114] Villanueva, Lozano H, Treviño Rangel RJ, González GM, Ramírez Elizondo MT, Lara Medrano R, et al. Outbreak of *Candida auris* infection in a COVID-19 hospital in Mexico. Clinical Microbiology and Infection. 2021;**27**(5): 813-816

[115] Ayala Gaytán JJ, Montoya AM, Martínez Resendez MF, Guajardo Lara CE, Treviño Rangel RdJ, Salazar Cavazos L, et al. First case of *Candida auris* isolated from the bloodstream of a Mexican patient with serious gastrointestinal complications from severe endometriosis. 2021;**49** (3):523-525. DOI: 10.1007/s15010-020-01525-1

[116] Pereira R, dosSantos Fontenelle RO, de Brito EHS, de Morais SM. Biofilm of Candida albicans: Formation, regulation and resistance. Journal of Applied Microbiology. 2021;**131**(1):11-22

[117] Khedri S, Santos ALS, Roudbary M, Hadighi R, Falahati M, Farahyar S, et al. Iranian HIV/AIDS patients with oropharyngeal candidiasis: Identification, prevalence and antifungal susceptibility of *Candida* species. Letters in Applied Microbiology. 2018;**67**(4):392-399

[118] Otašević S, Hay R. Superficial fungal infections. Frontiers in Cellular and Infection Microbiology. 2023;**11**: 1285771

[119] Alfaro-Alfaro N. Los determinantes sociales de la salud y las funciones esenciales de la salud pública social. Salud Jalisco. 2014;**1**(1):36-46

[120] OMS. Medidas Para Abordar Los Determinantes Sociales de la salud a fin de Promover la Equidad. Switzerland: COSUDE; 2021

[121] OMS. Equidad Sanitaria y Sus Determinantes. Switzerland: COSUDE; 2021

[122] Gaitán Cepeda LA, Sánchez Vargas LO, Pavia Ruz N, Muñoz Hernández R, Villegas Ham J, Caballos SA. Candida bucal en niños mexicanos con VIH/sida, desnutrición o marginación social. Revista Panamericana de Salud Pública. 2012;**31**(1):48-53

[123] Méndez Tovar LJ. Generalidades de las Micósis. In: López Martínez R, editor. Microbiología y Parasitología Médicas de Tay. 1.5th ed. Ciuad de México: Méndez Editores; 2019. pp. 856-858

[124] López-Martínez R, Ruiz-Sánchez D, Vértiz-Chávez E, Vaginal candidosis. Opportunistic factors and clinical correlation in 600 patients. Mycopathologia. 1984;**85**(3):167-170

[125] Spinillo A, Capuzzo E, Egbe Thomas O, Baltaro F, Nicola S, Piazzi G. Torulopsis glabrata Vaginitis. Obstetrics and Gynecology. 1995;**85**(6):993-998

[126] Laspina, Samudio M, Am C, Gm G, Ma B. Agentes Etiológicos de Vulvovaginitis en niñas. Memorias del Instituto de Investigaciones en Ciencias de la Salud. 2005;(3):9-14

[127] Lassey AT, Adanu RMK, Newman MJ, Opintah JA. Potential pathogens in the lower genital tract at manual vacuum aspiration for incomplete abortion in Korle Bu teaching hospital, Ghana. East African Medical Journal. 2004;**81**(8):398-401

[128] Patel V, Weiss HA, Mabey D, West B, D'Souza S, Patil V, et al. The burden and determinants of reproductive tract infections in India: A population based study of women in Goa, India. Sexually Transmitted Infections. 2006;**82**(3):243-249

[129] Torondel B, Sinha S, Mohanty JR, Swain T, Sahoo P, Panda B, et al. Association between unhygienic menstrual management practices and prevalence of lower reproductive tract infections: A hospital-based cross-sectional study in Odisha, India. BMC Infectious Diseases. 2018;**18**(1):1-12

[130] Na D, Weiping L, Enfeng Z, Chan W, Zhaozhao X, Honghui Z. Risk factors for Candida infection of the genital tract in the tropics. African Health Sciences. 2014;**14**(4):835-839

[131] Disha T, Haque F. Prevalence and risk factors of vulvovaginal Candidosis during pregnancy: A review. Infectious Diseases in Obstetrics and Gynecology. 2022;**2022**:1-14

[132] Duran Cañarte AL, Nicole Yuleidy AQ, Menéndez Gonzalez MG. Vaginal infections and risk factors in women of reproductive age: How much does it affect? Dom Cien. 2022;**8**(2): 289-309

[133] Marchaim D, Lemanek L, Bheemreddy S, Kaye KS, Sobel JD. Fluconazole-resistant candida albicans vulvovaginitis. Obstetrics and Gynecology. 2012;**120**(6):1407-1414

[134] Tavares Rodrigues M, Gonçalves AC, Tocantins Alvim MC, Castellano Filho DS, Barroso Zimmermmann J, da Silva VL, et al. Association between vaginal secretion culture, socio-demographic characteristics and clinical manifestations of patients with vulvovaginal candidiasis. Revista Brasileira de Ginecologia e Obstetrícia. 2013;**35**(12):554-561

[135] Wang DP, Lin RS. Epidemiologic differences between candidial and trichomonal infections as detected in cytologic smears in Taiwan. Public Health. 1995;**109**:443-450

[136] Atalaya R, Morales L. Prevalencia de candidiasis bucal en pacientes de la tercera edad que asisten a consulta médica al "hospital Jaime Mendoza" Sucre, enero-agosto del 2009. In: Ramos M, Pizarro J, Mojica M, Pereira N, Solis M, editors. Tópicos Selectos de Química. 1. Sucre: ECORFAN; 2014. pp. 298-331

[137] Domaneschi C, Massarente D, de Freitas R, de Sousa MH, Paula C, Migliari D, et al. Oral colonization by Candida species in AIDS pediatric

patients. Oral Diseases. 2011;**17**(4): 393-398

[138] Alkhars N, Zeng Y, Alomeir N, Al Jallad N, Wu TT, Aboelmagd S, et al. Oral Candida predicts Streptococcus mutans emergence in underserved US infants. Journal of Dental Research. 2022;**101**(1):54-62

[139] Moreira D, Palomari Spolidório DM, Rodrigues JAO, Boriollo MFG, Pereira CV, Rosa EA, et al. Candida spp. Biotypes in the Oral Cavity of School Children from Different Socioeconomic Categories in Piracicaba-SP, Brazil. Pesqui Odontol Bras. 2001;**15**(3):187-195

[140] Xiao J, Fogarty C, Wu TT, Alkhers N, Zeng Y, Thomas M, et al. Oral health and Candida carriage in socioeconomically disadvantaged US pregnant women. BMC Pregnancy and Childbirth. 2019;**19**(1):480

[141] Elangovan S, Srinivasan S, Allareddy V. Hospital-based emergency department visits with oral candidiasis in the USA. Oral Surgery, Oral Medicine, Oral Pathology and Oral Radiology. 2012;**114**(2):e26-e31

[142] Méndez, Tovar LJ, Anides Fonseca A, Vázquez Hernández A, Galindo González M, Díaz Madrid M, et al. Micosis observadas en cinco comunidades mexicanas con alto grado de marginación. Gaceta Médica de México. 2006;**142**(5):381-386

[143] Almendros De Oliveira AJ, De Aguiar BJ, Alves Cortez AC, De Oliveira RL, SJ. Superficial mycoses in the City of Manaus/AM between march and November/2003. Anais Brasileiros de Dermatologia. 2006;**81**(3):238-281

[144] Durkin MJ, Dukes JL, Reeds DN, Mazuski JE, Camins BC. A descriptive study of the risk factors associated with catheter-related bloodstream infections in the home parenteral nutrition population. Journal of Parenteral and Enteral Nutrition. 2016;**40**(7):1006-1013

[145] Klufio CA, Amoa AB, Delamare O, Hombhanje M, Kariwiga G, Igo J. Prevalence of vaginal infections with bacterial vaginosis, trichomonas vaginalis and Candida albicans among pregnant women at the Port Moresby general hospital antenatal clinic. Papua and New Guinea Medical Journal. 1995; **38**(3):163-171

[146] Gertig DM, Kapiga SH, Shao JF, Hunter DJ. Risk factors for sexually transmitted diseases among women attending family planning clinics in Dar-es-salaam, Tanzania. Sexually Transmitted Infections. 1997;**73**(1):39-43

[147] Medina R, Mella L, Espoz H, Medina E, Cumsille F. Prostitutes of the east sector of Santiago: Characteristics and pathology of sexual transmission. Revista medica de Chile. 1989;**117**(9): 1063-1067

[148] Souza PC, Storti-Filho A, Souza RJS, Damke E, Mello ICJ, Pereira MW, et al. Prevalence of Candida sp. in the cervical-vaginal cytology stained by Harris-Shorr. Archives of Gynecology and Obstetrics. 2009;**279**(5): 625-629

[149] López-Monteon A, Gómez-Figueroa FS, Ramos-Poceros G, Guzmán-Gómez D, Ramos-Ligonio A. Codetection of trichomonas vaginalis and Candida albicans by PCR in urine samples in a low-risk population attended in a clinic first level in Central Veracruz, Mexico. BioMed Research International. 2013;**2013**:281892

[150] Akoh CC, Pressman EK, Cooper E, Queenan RA, Pillittere J, O'Brien KO. Prevalence and risk factors for infections

in a pregnant adolescent population. Journal of Pediatric and Adolescent Gynecology. 2017;**30**(1):71-75

[151] Valencia Arredondo M, Yepes López WA. Prevalencia y factores asociados con vaginosis bacterianas, candidiasis y tricomoniasis en dos hospitales de los municipios de Apartadó y Rionegro -Antioquia, 2014. IATREIA. 2018;**31**(2):133-144

[152] Shazadi K, Liaqat I, Tajammul A, Mehreen A, Arshad N. Comparison and association between different types of vaginitis and risk factors among reproductive aged women in Lahore, Pakistan: A cross-sectional study. Brazilian Archives of Biology and Technology. 2022;**65**:1-10

[153] Eidt G, Waltermann EDM, Hilgert JB, Arthur RA. Candida and dental caries in children, adolescents and adults: A systematic review and meta-analysis. Archives of Oral Biology. 2020; **119**:104876

[154] Cobos Lladó D, Fierro Arias L, Arellano Mendoza I, Bonifaz A. Onychomycosis and its influence on quality life. Dermatología Cosmética, Médica y Quirúrgica. 2016;**14**(4):318-327

Section 3

Antifungal Drugs and Nanomaterials

Chapter 5

Antifungal Resistance in *Candida albicans*

Simasadat Seyedjavadi, Farahnaz Hatami and Zahra Jahanshiri

Abstract

Candidiasis can present as an infection in the skin, mucous membranes, or deep-seated organs, caused by various types of *Candida* spp. *C. albicans* is one of the most prevalent *Candida* spp. causing diseases. These yeasts typically inhabit the normal human microbiota. High-risk individuals include those with cancer, diabetes, HIV/AIDS, and organ transplants. Due to the similarity between fungi and their human hosts as eukaryotes, the potential molecular targets for developing antifungal treatments are limited. This poses a significant health concern as drug resistance becomes increasingly prevalent. Currently, only four main classes of approved antifungal agents are used for treating *invasive fungal infections:* azoles, echinocandins, polyenes, and 5-fluorocytosine (5-FC). These antifungals inhibit different biosynthetic pathways in various pathogenic fungi. For instance, echinocandins focus on cell wall biosynthesis, while azoles, together with allylamines, inhibit ergosterol biosynthesis, and 5-flucytosine (5-FC) targets DNA, RNA, and protein synthesis. Azole antifungal agents are widely used as therapeutic options for the treatment of fungal infections, but their fungistatic nature leads to the evolution of *C. albicans* resistance to azole. In addition to azoles, *C. albicans* also develop resistance to polyenes, echinocandins, and 5-FC. This chapter provides a detailed discussion on the mechanisms of action and mechanisms involved in *Candida albicans* antifungal drug resistance.

Keywords: antifungal, *Candida albicans*, resistance, azoles, polyenes, echinocandins, 5-flucytosine, biofilm

1. Introduction

Candida spp. are typically harmless and normally live on human skin, gastrointestinal, and genital tracts. However, in certain individuals such as the elderly, hospitalized patients, or those with weakened immune systems, *Candida* is capable of inducing a range of infections. Indeed, *Candida* fungal infections are the most prevalent human fungal disease globally [1]. The most frequently isolated species in clinical cases are *C. albicans* (37%) and *C. glabrata* (27%). Other species commonly found in bloodstream infections include *C. krusei*, *C. dubliniensis*, *C. parapsilosis*, *C. lusitaniae*, *C. tropicalis*, and the more recently emerging *C. auris*. *C. auris* is particularly concerning as it is resistant to multiple drugs, often misidentified, and poses a significant threat in healthcare settings [2]. According to the CDC (Centers for Disease Control and Prevention) *reports*, approximately 34,000 cases of candidiasis were observed among patients admitted to a hospital in 2017, resulting in about 1700 deaths [3]. Candidiasis encompasses a wide range of clinical presentations, from relatively mild mucocutaneous infections to severe invasive diseases such as candidemia, with mortality rates ranging from 30% to 47% [4]. Medical device-associated infections such as *vascular catheters*, cardiovascular devices, *central venous catheter*, and urinary catheters are commonly associated with *Candida* infections [5]. Candidemia, in particular, can lead to the dissemination of the infection to various organs [6]. Due to the lack of rapid and sensitive diagnostic tests for invasive *Candida* infections, the majority of cases are detected using routine culture-based methods. The sensitivity of this method may be restricted and can sometimes produce false-positive results due to contamination during the process [7]. In the intensive care unit, febrile or septic patients with a central venous catheter (CVC) who have recently undergone abdominal surgery or chemotherapy often receive empiric antifungal therapy when antimicrobial therapy fails to respond [8]. However, this approach can lead to the inappropriate use of antifungal drugs and the development of resistance in people without infections, or it can lead to the postponement of effective treatment for people who are truly infected [2]. The treatment approach for invasive *Candida* infections depends on various factors, including the host's *immune* response, as well as the severity and location of the infection [9]. Besides implementing appropriate source control measures, removal of contaminated medical devices and administering antifungal drugs have proven to be crucial therapeutic approaches in the management of *Candida* infections [10].

Currently, the most commonly used antifungals that are effective against *Candida* spp., are azoles, polyenes, 5-flucytosine, and echinocandins [11]. Compared to the emergence of antimicrobial resistance in infections caused by bacteria, the development of antifungal resistance in *Candida* spp. is a global public health threat. The main objective of this chapter is to provide a detailed explanation of the mechanisms through which these antifungals exert their effects, in addition to outlining the strategies employed by *Candida* spp. to acquire resistance to these drugs.

2. The targets of antifungals

Candidiasis can be effectively managed through the use of antifungal medications from various drug classes that act on distinct cellular processes, resulting in either growth inhibition (fungistatic) or cell death (fungicidal) of the yeast pathogens. These cellular processes encompass the synthesis of the *plasma* membrane, cell wall, and RNA. Every one of these processes encompasses a series of enzymatic reactions [2]. The subsequent section provides an overview of the targets and mode of action of antifungals utilized for candidiasis treatment.

2.1 Antifungals that target ergosterol and ergosterol biosynthesis

Antifungal medications that specifically target ergosterol and its biosynthesis play a crucial role in the treatment of fungal infections. Ergosterol is an essential component of cell membranes in fungi and it is critical for maintaining the integrity and functionality of the *membranes* of fungi. Additionally, ergosterol and sphingolipids participate *in* the formation specialized *lipid rafts*. Lipid rafts harbor numerous biologically significant proteins that participate in diverse cellular functions, including signaling, stress-response, and nutrient transportation [12, 13]. The biosynthesis of ergosterol relies on a series of 25 distinct enzymatic reactions. This biosynthetic pathway provides an attractive drug target because ergosterol is essential for fungi, whereas it is absent in humans. Consequently, several drugs have been designed to inhibit the synthesis of this fungal lipid or directly target ergosterol itself, and the following section provides a detailed description of these.

2.1.1 Azoles

Azoles are a class of antifungal compounds characterized by a five-membered heterocyclic structure. Two subgroups exist within the azole group of antifungal drugs: imidazoles and triazoles. In the azole ring, imidazoles (ketoconazole, clotrimazole, miconazole, tioconazole, and econazole) contain two nitrogen atoms while triazoles (voriconazole, fluconazole, itraconazole, posaconazole, and isavuconazole) contain three nitrogen atoms. Ketoconazole, which has become the standard medication for treating candidiasis and infections caused by dimorphic fungi, is known to be associated with notable liver toxicity. Fluconazole is the most frequently employed in therapeutic applications [14].

Second generation of triazoles, with broad-spectrum antifungal activity, include voriconazole (VOR), posaconazole (POS), and isavuconazole (ISV). These antifungal agents exhibit increased potency against resistant *pathogenic fungi*. Isavuconazole, in particular, is a new broad-spectrum triazole that demonstrates comparable efficacy to voriconazole but with reduced toxicity. The lower toxicity of isavuconazole can be attributed to its high water solubility. Azoles are *used* as commercial *antifungals* for the prevention and treatment of *Candida* infections. They are inhibitors of the sterol *14-α-demethylase enzyme* (ERG11 in yeast), which plays a crucial role in the ergosterol synthesis pathway [15]. Azols bind to Erg11 and thereby block the production of ergosterol in the fungal cell membrane. Additionally, azoles have the ability to increase reactive oxygen species (ROS) production [16].

2.1.1.1 Azole drug resistance

Over the course of many years, there has been significant research exploring the molecular bases underlying the mechanisms of resistance of pathogenic fungi to azole drugs. The subsequent sections will outline the distinct mechanisms that contribute to azole resistance.

2.1.1.2 Overexpression of cell membrane efflux pumps

The overexpression of efflux pumps in the plasma membrane is a significant mechanism that controls *resistance to azole* in various fungal pathogens [17]. The primary group of efflux pumps linked with resistance to azoles are ABC transporters (ATP-binding cassettes). ABC transporters comprise two membrane-spanning domains (MSD) and two nucleotide-binding domains (NBDs). The NBD uses *ATP* energy and transfer of substrates across membranes [18]. Another important efflux pump is the main facilitator (MF) superfamily associated with azole resistance. MF transporters, like the ABC superfamily, have transmembrane-spanning helices. However, instead of relying on ATP, MF transporters employ the proton gradient across the plasma membrane to facilitate the movement of substrates [19, 20].

In *C. albicans*, upregulation of two closely related ABC transporters, *CDR1* and *CDR2*, is related to resistance to azole, especially in patients receiving prolonged antifungal therapy [21, 22]. Among these transporters, *CDR1* plays a primary role in azole resistance, as removing *CDR1* from a clinical strain reduces azole resistance by 4- to 8-fold. On the other hand, the deletion of *CDR2* generally has a lesser effect [23]. The *Tac1* functions as a transcription factor of *CDR* and binds to specific DREs (drug-response elements) in both the *CDR1* and *CDR2* promoters, regulating their expression. Notably, the mutated Tac1 alleles lead to overexpression of both *CDR1* and *CDR2,* which is associated with azole resistance [24].

Although the *C. albicans* genome encodes 95 MF transporters, resistance to fluconazole is associated only with multidrug resistance 1 (Mdr1) [25, 26]. The *transcription factor* Mrr1 controls *MDR1* efflux *pump expression* and mediates *multidrug resistance* in *C. albicans*. Inactivation *of MRR1* in *fluconazole-resistant C. albicans* leads to loss of *MDR1 expression* and *increased fluconazole susceptibility*, whereas activating point mutations in *MRR1* enhances azole resistance [27, 28]. A *recent* study demonstrated that the Swi/Snf chromatin remodeling complex in *C. albicans* has been identified as coactivator of *MRR1*. Interestingly, genetic inactivation of *SNF2*, the *catalytic subunit* of *Swi/Snf*, significantly reduces the upregulation of *MDR1* expression and resistance to fluconazole [29].

2.1.1.3 Changes in targets of drug

In *C. albicans*, the development of azole resistance frequently involves substitutions of amino acids in the drug target Erg11, resulting in a diminished binding affinity between the lanosterol demethylase enzyme and the drug. These substitutions are primarily concentrated in specific regions of *Erg11*, including amino acids 105–165, 266–287, and 405–488 [30]. Although more than 140 amino acid substitutions in *Erg11* have been related to azole resistance, only a limited number of these substitutions have been shown experimentally to induce resistance [31]. Molecular mapping of *C. albicans ERG11* variants has revealed that these mutations are located in crucial areas such as the enzyme's catalytic site, the unique external loop found in fungi [32].

In azole-resistant clinical isolates of *C. albicans*, there is a prevalent occurrence of *ERG11* overexpression, directly contributing to an increased abundance of the drug target and subsequently reducing drug susceptibility [21, 22]. The transcriptional activator *Upc2* plays a critical role in regulating several genes involved in ergosterol biosynthesis, including *ERG11*, in *C. albicans* [33, 34].

2.1.1.4 Stress-response modulation

Fungal pathogens inhabit diverse and ever-changing environments that are prone to fluctuations in temperature, pH, and nutrient availability. These fluctuations can disrupt the normal balance within fungal cells and impose significant stress. The presence of antifungal agents further adds to this stress, and fungal pathogens in order to survive, need to identify, adapt, and respond to the stress imposed by antifungal drugs. Therefore, pathogenic fungi have developed extensive stress-response mechanisms that enable them to grow despite various cellular challenges [35].

One notable mechanism by which *C. albicans* develops azole resistance is through modifications in the ergosterol biosynthesis pathway, which is associated with stress responses [36]. Specifically, mutations in the *ERG3* gene prevent the accumulation of a toxic sterol intermediate that allows the *continuation* of the reproduction and growth of the fungi in the *presence* of azoles. The presence of these mutations is associated with resistance to azole drugs in *C. albicans* [37].

Hsp90 (*heat shock protein 90*) is a crucial regulator of stress responses in fungal pathogens [38]. It interacts with various cochaperones to recognize specific client proteins involved in regulatory networks [39]. Hsp90 acts as a reservoir for storing and releasing genetic variation, as well as an enhancer that facilitates the rapid emergence of new traits [40]. In the case of *C. albicans*, Hsp90 is involved in the evolution of resistance to azole. Nonetheless, in *C. albicans* isolates where resistance arises from the overexpression of efflux pumps, Hsp90 does not serve as a mediator of azole resistance, suggesting the presence of an autonomous resistance mechanism [41].

Hsp90 enables the resistance of various fungi against drugs that target the cell membrane and cell wall, and calcineurin is the main mediator of Hsp90-dependent azole resistance [42]. In *C. albicans*, azole treatment induces a calcineurin-dependent stress-response, and disruption of this phosphatase makes *C. albicans* highly sensitive to azoles [41]. Blocking Hsp90 activity prevents the activation of the calcineurin-dependent stress-response by azoles [43].

Protein kinase C (Pkc1) and other kinases also play a role in the stress-response mechanism that allows *C. albicans* to survive azole-induced stress. Disrupting PKC-MAPK signaling reduces azole resistance in different clinical isolates of *C. albicans* [44]. Additionally, kinases such as casein kinase 2 (CK2) and target of rapamycin (TOR) kinases are involved in azole resistance. Inhibiting TOR function eliminates *erg3*-mediated resistance to azoles [45].

Post-translational modifications are important in regulating the stress-response pathway *and alter virulence in an antifungal drug-dependent manner* in *Candida* spp. [46]. Lysine acetyl-transferases (KATs) and lysine deacetylases (KDACs) play a significant role in chromatin-mediated transcription and the post-translational control of cellular proteins. Suppression of these enzymes leads to resistance to antifungal medications [47].

2.1.1.5 Modifications of genome

Fungi have the ability to adapt genetically to their environment and develop resistance to antifungal therapies. This adaptability is achieved through significant genetic modifications, including aneuploidies, loss of heterozygosity (LOH), and rearrangements of chromosomes [48]. Aneuploidy, in particular, allows fungi to quickly acquire diverse characteristics without permanently committing to the mutant genotype [49]. Fungistatic azoles induce changes in DNA content and cell morphology, favoring the formation of aneuploidy [50]. Chromosome 5 in *C. albicans* is commonly affected by an isochromosome [i(5L)], which is associated with azole resistance. The resistance is attributed to amplified quantities of *ERG11* and *TAC1*, mutations that enhance functionality, and loss of heterozygosity (LOH) in these determinants [51–53]. Experimental evolution studies have shown that strains acquiring resistance to azoles exhibit extensive aneuploidies, particularly involving chromosome 4 [53]. LOH events can also impact drug resistance, which is commonly observed in genomic regions containing susceptibility determinants. LOH can generate hyperactive alleles, leading to increased expression of genes involved in drug resistance [27]. Stress conditions can elevate mitotic recombination rates in *C. albicans*, resulting in increased LOH rates [54]. These findings propose a potential mechanism by which *C. albicans* can achieve increased genetic variation in response to environmental disruptions, given its absence of a traditional sexual reproduction cycle.

2.1.1.6 Intrinsic resistance to antifungals

Until now, our research has primarily focused on comprehending the development of resistance to antifungal agents in fungal pathogens. However, it is crucial to acknowledge that certain fungi inherently possess resistance to commonly used antifungals. Investigating the mechanisms underlying intrinsic resistance is essential for obtaining a better understanding of the clinical consequences caused by fungal pathogens. Intrinsic resistance has also been observed in specific non-*albicans Candida* (NCA) spp., particularly toward azole drugs [55]. For example, *C. glabrata* exhibits substantial resistance to fluconazole even in the absence of prior exposure to the drug [56]. This resistance is mainly attributed to the increased expression of specific ABC transporters regulated by the transcription factor *Pdr1* [57].

In addition, antifungal resistance can be inherent to different growth states of common nonresistant fungal spp. [58]. In the natural environments, *Candida* spp. often grow as biofilms, densely packed *communities* of cells *adhered* to *a surface* [59]. Among fungal pathogens, *C. albicans* can form biofilms on medical devices and host tissue. *C. albicans* planktonic cells do not have intrinsic resistance to antifungal agents, but *C. albicans biofilms are intrinsically resistant* to conventional *antifungal* [60].

Cells within these biofilms *overexpressed efflux pumps* and efflux*genes CDR1* and *MDR1*, which contribute to strong azole resistance [61]. The synthesis of glucan by *Fks1* is a known mechanism that contributes to *C. albicans* biofilm antifungal drug resistance [62]. This resistance mechanism was observed in azoles, polyenes, and echinocandins.

2.1.2 Polyenes

Polyenes are fungicidal *medications* that target ergosterol in the fungal *cell membrane* and initiate cell lysis [63]. They bind with ergosterol and *form pores in the cell membrane* that cause *rapid leakage of monovalent ions* such as potassium (K^+), sodium (Na^+), hydrogen (H^+), and chloride (Cl^-), ultimately leading to cell death in *fungi* [14]. The *polyene* antifungals *include amphotericin B* and *nystatin.* Despite the introduction of various new antifungal agents, particularly the second-generation triazoles and the echinocandins, *amphotericin B* remains the predominant and crucially important drug in the management of severe systemic fungal infections [64, 65]. Amphotericin B is rarely necessary for the management of invasive candidiasis, as it is typically reserved for cases where the *Candida* spp., exhibits resistance to alternative drug classes.

2.1.2.1 Mechanism of action

2.1.2.1.1 Polyene-Sterol interaction

Overall, the activity of polyenes compared to other classes of antifungals is different and not usual, as they interact with ergosterol as a vital molecule instead of targeting a specific enzyme [66]. So, polyene antibiotics mainly affect ergosterol and ergosterol biosynthetic pathways [67, 68]. Currently, there are four models for describing the activity of the polyene antifungal including the model of polyenes forming ion-leaking pores in the membrane, the polyene-Ergosterol adsorption at the surface model, the sterol sponge model, and the oxidative damage model, which binding to ergosterol (an important component in fungi, which is responsible for different processes in the cell, namely: the membrane proteins regulation, endocytosis, division of cells, signaling of the cell and fluidity of the membrane [69]) plays an important role to its antifungal effect in every proposed model [70]. Three interactive forces contribute to the binding of AmB and ergosterol. Van der Waals forces, network of hydrogen bonds, and π–π electronic interactions [69].

2.1.2.1.2 Pore-forming models

In the mechanism of forming pore, which is the most studied one, an ion channel-like complex is formed from the interaction between polyenes and ergosterol, which leads to the release of some ions and small molecules from the inner plasma membrane to the out and eventually leads to cell destruction. In light of the amphipathic nature of polyenes, they would position themselves within the phospholipid bilayer in such a way that the hydrophobic polyene "tail" interacts with ergosterol, and on the other side, the hydrophilic "head" participates in forming an aqueous channel. Typically, a pore is made from the gathering of 4–12 polyene monomers [70]. The first channel is formed by one cylindrical ring of AmB-ergosterol complexes that is placed on another ring and is named the "complete-pore" channel. The second one is just composed of one cylindrical ring known as the "half-pore" channel.

These channels have nearly equal length as membrane phospholipids, on average, both types are essentially the same in structure, but the second type makes the lipid bilayer structure thinner. The formation of pores depends on three factors: primarily polyene and later composition of the membrane as well as its thickness [71]. In a membrane composed mostly of dimyristoylphosphatidylcholine (DMPC), for instance, AmB would mainly create half-pores [72].

2.1.2.1.3 Surface adsorption and sterols Sponge models

Recent studies have demonstrated that the fungicidal activity of AmB is not solely dependent on ion channel formation, but rather, glycosylation-dependent ergosterol sequestration has been identified as essential [73]. In the "surface adsorption model," polyenes can lead to the movement of ergosterol molecules and absorb them toward the surface of the phospholipid membrane [69]. In light of this hypothesis, in the "sterol sponge" mode of action that Anderson and his colleagues proposed, AmB molecules are positioned parallelly in a large-extra membranous aggregate and extract the ergosterols from the membrane [74].

In the second and third models both, by absorbing or extracting ergosterol from the membrane, the bilayer of phospholipids becomes unstable and eventually, leads to disruption in vital cellular activities [71] and, eventually, cell death [74]. Anderson also proposes that the primary toxic factor of AmB toward mammalian cells is caused by the formation of these large aggregates of AmB-ergosterol at the outside of the membrane. Hence, the production of better antifungal derivatives by making the binding of the drug to ergosterol as effective as possible could significantly enhance its therapeutic efficacy [70].

2.1.2.1.4 Other proposed modes of action

Alterations in the permeability and disturbances of the membrane might be attributed to the amphotericin B fungicidal effects; however, its lethal effects cannot be explained [75]. The precise mechanism behind the occurrence of oxidative stress remains unclear. Nevertheless, one suggested explanation is that the binding of polyenes to the membrane initiates a response leading to the generation of reactive oxygen species (ROS), such as hydrogen peroxide (H_2O_2), superoxide ($-O_2$), and hydroxyl radicals, which modifies the main macromolecules such as DNA, proteins and lipids and finally causes membrane instability and cell death. Therefore, there is a correlation between ROS production with apoptosis and aging [69, 75–77].

Alternatively, it is possible that the antifungal agent itself can auto-oxidize and start the oxidative stress process [69]. However, ROS production can be limited by catalase activity owing to its antioxidant characteristic during AmB therapy which leads to cell protection [78, 79].

2.1.2.2 Polyene drug resistance

The incidence of polyene resistance in isolated fungal strains is relatively low. As far as the susceptibility rate to this antifungal among some Candida species, such as *C. albicans, C. glabrata*, and *C. parapsilosis*, is reported to be nearly 100% in surveillance studies [80]. However, various mechanisms of action for describing how resistance occurs have been stated. Amphotericin B resistance is most likely to be acquired through the changes in the sterol composition of the fungal cell phospholipid layer, which is attributed to being the most frequent mechanism [69]. This change is often linked to a general rise in membrane sterol levels and changes in phospholipids, leading to alterations in the quantity or quality of sterol content within the cell. These changes eventually affect the amount or availability of ergosterol for the polyenes' activity [81]. The mechanism has been associated with various mutations in genes responsible for biosynthesis pathways of ergosterol, particularly those found in *ERG1* to *ERG6* and *ERG11* genes [82, 83]. It has been demonstrated that the absence of *ERG11* and *ERG3* gene activity, as an example, in *C. albicans* results in the replacement of ergosterol with other sterols such as lanosterol, eburicol, and 4,14-dimethyl-zymosterol in the membrane [69]. Besides genetic modifications, treatment with azole antifungals has been linked to an increased resistance level to polyenes in *Candida* species due to the reduction in cellular ergosterol levels caused by azole [83].

Getting protected against oxidative damage is another factor in developing resistance to amphotericin B [84]. Therefore, the second hypothesis is that, the reactive oxygen species (ROS) generated owing to exposure to AmB, can be broken down and result in toleration to the induced oxidative stress by polyene. This is accomplished through catalase activity, Hsp90 and Hsp70 (the molecular chaperones of the heat shock protein (HSP) family) [82]. Evidence has illustrated that decreased fatal consequences of AmB on protoplasts and *C. albicans* result from a rise in the catalase intracellular or extracellular levels, as well as hypoxic conditions incubation [84]. The fitness and survival of Candida isolates that are resistant to amphotericin B, are highly reliant on the expression and functionality of Hsp90. By inhibiting Hsp90 pharmacologically, in *C. albicans* or *C. tropicalis* strains resistant to AmB, the resistance completely disappeared [85]. Moreover, the modifications in cell wall structure and the fungal cell's growth phase may be associated with polyene resistance [79].

Several studies have indicated that certain cell wall components are implicated in the cell's resistance to amphotericin B. For instance, in *C. albicans* a reduced level of chitin has been observed with increased resistance to amphotericin B. Moreover, the production of glucan may increase due to regulatory mechanisms influenced by exposure to or resistance against AmB, which might physically obstruct the entry of AmB into the cell wall [86]. The exact function of glucans in the cell wall, which blocks amphotericin B's ability to access ergosterol and plays a role in resistance, is still unclear [75].

During the logarithmic growth phase, there is a higher rate of cell wall degradation and resynthesis. This increased activity allows enhanced access of amphotericin B to the cell membrane. This process, in the stationary growth phase, is found at a much lower rate, which results in the creation of relative resistance to amphotericin B [81].

2.2 Antifungals that target biosynthesis of the cell wall

In addition to ergosterol in *Candida* spp., the biosynthesis of the fungal cell wall is also a target for the development of new antifungal therapies [87]. The fungal cell wall is a rigid layer around the plasma membrane of fungal cells that defends against osmotic stress. The structure *of* the *cell wall* is unique to *fungi*, and since it is absent in humans, an *associated enzyme* in cell wall *biosynthesis* is a promising *target* for *antifungal drug* [88].

2.2.1 Echinocandin

Echinocandins, such as caspofungin, micafungin, and anidulafungin, specifically target the cell wall. Echinocandin B, the initial antifungal drug of this class, was discovered in the 1970s and exhibited effective antifungal properties, albeit with hemolytic activity. To mitigate this effect, cilofungin was synthesized. However, this compound was withdrawn because of its low water solubility and co-solvent toxicity. Subsequently, two compounds, pneumocandin A and pneumocandin B, were identified during the echinocandin research process. In 1992, caspofungin acetate was synthesized from pneumocandin B, receiving approval from the US Food and Drug Administration (FDA) in January 2001. Micafungin, which demonstrated low hemolytic activity and potency on *Candida* spp., was permitted in the United States in 2005 and in Europe in 2008. This agent was also accepted for the treatment of aggressive candidiasis. Further refinement of the chemical construction of echinocandin B led to the development of anidulafungin, which obtained US approval in 2006 [89].

2.2.2 Mechanisms of action

Echinocandins belong to a group of antifungal agents that impact the fungal cell wall by inhibiting the activity of UDP-glucose (1,3)-D-glucan-β-(3)-D-glucosyltransferase. This enzyme plays a crucial role in synthesizing β-(1,3-D)-glucan, a vital component of the cell walls in numerous fungi, within the glucan biosynthesis pathway [90], and disrupt the integrity and shape of the cell wall. They are structurally defined by a cyclic hexapeptide core attached to a lipid side chain of variable configuration [91]. These antifungals act by non-competitive inhibition of the synthesis of 1,3-α-D-glucan in fungi [90]. Currently, echinocandins are the recommended initial treatment for candidemia and other forms of invasive candidiasis [92]. Echinocandins are considered the primary therapy for candidemia. The development of echinocandin resistance in *Candida* spp. is predominantly linked to acquiring *FKS* mutations [93].

2.2.3 Echinocandin drug resistance

Fungi employ adaptive strategies to compete with other microorganisms within their ecological niche and obtain necessary resources. As an important part of these adaptations, the emergence of antifungal drug resistance is possible [94]. The resistance mechanism of echinocandins involves alterations in specific amino acid regions known as "hot spots" within the *FKS*-encoded subunits of glucan synthase. These alterations reduce the enzyme's sensitivity to the drug and result in higher minimum inhibitory concentration (MIC) values [95]. These changes can lead to elevated MIC values. In *C. albicans,* Ser641 and Ser645 are the most reported amino acid alterations that pronounced resistance phenotype [96].

2.2.4 MIC values, medicinal use, and effective dose

Micafungin demonstrates strong antifungal efficacy against a wide spectrum of *Candida* spp., including those that exhibit resistance to azoles, amphotericin B, and other echinocandins [97]. **Table 1** displays the breakpoint values for echinocandins, including anidulafungin (AND), caspofungin (CAS), and micafungin (MCF), alongside *Candida albicans*, as determined by both the Clinical and Laboratory Standards Institute (CLSI) and the European Committee for Antimicrobial Susceptibility Testing (EUCAST) [99]. It has been reported that in anidulafungin-resistant *C. albicans* isolates, the presence of mutations in the *FKS* gene confirms resistance to MCF. Due to significant discrepancies across laboratories, the breakpoints for caspofungin remain unknown [98].

2.3 Antifungals that target nucleic acid biosynthesis

Medications that focus on the synthesis of nucleic acids play a crucial role in the effective management of fungal infections and have been utilized since the 1950s. Among these antifungal agents is 5-flucytosine (5FC), which hampers both fungal protein synthesis and DNA replication by integrating into RNA. The entry of 5-FC into fungal cells occurs via the cytosine permease enzyme [100]. When 5FC enters the cell, it is converted to 5-fluorouracil (5FU), which undergoes further metabolic processes to form 5-fluorouridine triphosphate (5FUTP). Instead of uridine triphosphate (UTP), 5FUTP is incorporated into fungal RNA, leading to alteration of tRNA

Antifungal agents	Standard	*C. albicans*	
		S≤	R>
AND	EUCAST	0.03	0.03
	CLSI	0.25	0.5
CAS	EUCAST	N	N
	CLSI	0.25	0.5
MCF	EUCAST	0.016	0.016
	CLSI	0.25	0.5

N—until caspofungin breakpoints have been established, the susceptibility of this echinocandin should be considered based on the susceptibility of the remaining two echinocandins. So, if the isolate is susceptible to anidulafungin as well as micafungin, it should be considered susceptible to caspofungin.

Table 1.
Breakpoints of echinocandins proven by CLSI and EUCAST [98].

and disruption of protein synthesis and growth inhibition. An alternative metabolic transformation of 5FU involves its conversion to 5-Fluorodeoxyuridine monophosphate (5FdUMP), which functions as a potent inhibitor of thymidylate synthase. This enzyme plays a vital role in the biosynthesis of DNA [100].

2.3.1 Flucytosine

Flucytosine, also referred to as 5-fluorocytosine (5-FC), is an antifungal medication primarily used in combination with amphotericin B for the treatment of severe fungal infections [101]. However, the clinical utility of 5-FC is hampered by the frequent occurrence of both primary and acquired resistance, particularly when administered as a standalone therapy. Previous investigations have predominantly focused on elucidating resistance mechanisms in S. *cerevisiae* and *C. albicans*, with a specific emphasis on mutations affecting key enzymes involved in the pyrimidine salvage pathways [102, 103]. Studies have revealed that resistance to 5-FC can arise through the inactivation or modification of various enzymes responsible for activating cytosine permease, cytosine deaminase, or uracil phosphoribosyl transferase, as well as through an increase in pyrimidine production [104]. Nevertheless, the absence of mutations in these enzymes among clinically resistant isolates suggests the existence of additional regulatory mechanisms within fungal cells. Despite the fact that resistance to 5-FC can develop in a single step, its progression can occur rapidly regardless of the dosage or site of infection when used as a monotherapy [104].

The prevalence of *Candida* spp., which exhibits primary 5-FC resistance is less than 5%, with the exception of *C. krusei*, which exhibits resistance in approximately 35% of isolates [105]. The emergence of resistance in *Candida* is influenced by a multitude of factors including species, clade, genotype, ploidy, and the presence of a phenotype mutator [106]. The reported range of 5-FC resistance in *C. albicans* is 0 to 3% [107]. In *C. albicans*, the uptake of 5FC is facilitated by the cytosine permease, CaFcy2p, which is subsequently transformed into 5FU through the action of cytosine deaminase, CaFcy1p [108]. The conversion of 5FU to 5FUMP is accomplished by the phosphoribosyl transferase, CaFur1p. Disruption or inactivation of these enzymes leads to an elevated resistance to 5FC. Estrella et al. observed a correlation between resistance to 5-FC and a decreased susceptibility to azoles [106]. Additionally, Dodgson et al. identified a single alteration in the *FUR1* gene, resulting in an amino acid substitution, which is associated with a reduced susceptibility or increased resistance to 5-FC [109].

3. *Candida* biofilms and resistance

Biofilm alludes to a collective gathering of cells that adhere to one another and are surrounded by an exopolysaccharide matrix. The properties of biofilms are different from planktonic cells [110]. These biofilms may be made by either only one species or multiple species [111]. Research has shown that biofilms are responsible for over 80% of all microbial infections [112]. During the initial stage of biofilm formation, yeast cells adhere to a surface, leading to the development of separated colonies. This is followed by an intermediate phase where yeast cells produce and secrete extracellular polymeric substances (EPS) [113]. The extracellular matrix, which comprises proteins (55%), carbohydrates (25%), lipids (15%), and extracellular DNA (5%), has been found to play a significant role in antifungal resistance [114]. The maturation and three-dimensional structure of the *Candida* biofilm are facilitated by these compounds [115]. The main specification of biofilms is dependent on the *Candida* spp., [116]. The biofilm structure contributes to difficult treatment and a high range of morbidity and mortality [117]. The matrix supports the whole construction of biofilm and acts as a physical obstacle to drug diffusion. Moreover, in the matrix of biofilms, Mannan and glucan plays important role in arresting antifungals and increasing the resistance of the biofilm to antifungals, in relation to planktonic cells [118]. In 1995, Hawser and Douglas provided the initial evidence of antifungal resistance in *Candida* biofilm, specifically in *C. albicans*, marking a significant milestone in the field [119]. Studies have demonstrated that drug resistance in biofilm has several causes, such as penetration of high-density cells, decrease of the growth rate, nutrient restriction, extracellular matrix formation, existence of persister cells, gene expression changes, and increase of sterol content in *Candida* cell layer [116].

3.1 Cell density and growth limitation

The resistance of *Candida* biofilms to antifungal agents is influenced by the concentration ratio of *Candida* cells within the biofilm structure, which is significantly higher compared to planktonic cells [120]. The biofilm structure of *C. albicans* typically consists of two distinct layers: a thin basal yeast layer and a thicker, densely packed hyphal layer [121]. These characteristics are correlated with a common resistance to antifungal triazoles and/or amphotericin B [122]. Moreover, it has been observed that the cells located in more profound layers of the biofilm, because of nutrient scarcity, exhibit slower growth and consequently develop higher resistance to antifungal drugs.

3.2 Extracellular matrix production

The extracellular matrix (ECM) present in *Candida* biofilms serves as a protective barrier, shielding the biofilm cells from detrimental factors such as antifungal agents and host immune responses [123]. Research has indicated that the chemical structure of the ECM not only hinders diffusion and penetration but also contributes to the development of resistance. It has been reported that DNA has an important role in the biofilm formation of *C. albicans*, structural integrity, and enhanced efficacy of echinocandins and polyenes [121]. Additionally, β-1,3 glucans, which are the predominant carbohydrate constituents of the biofilm, are responsible for sequestering azoles, echinocandins, pyrimidines, and polyenes within *C. albicans* biofilms [115]. Studies have revealed that the *SMI1* gene plays a role in cell wall glucans, ECM production, and drug resistance. This gene functions through the transcription factor Rlmp and the glucan synthase *FKS1* [122]. Furthermore, the zinc-response transcription factor *ZAP1* acts as a negative regulator of the soluble β-1,3 glucan ECM in *C. albicans* biofilms [123]. Gca1 and Gca2 have positive roles in matrix production, while ADH5, CSH1, and LFD6, a group of alcohol dehydrogenases, also contribute to matrix production, with CSH1 and LFD6 having negative effects and ADH5 having a positive effect [115].

3.3 Presence of Persister cells

Within a biofilm, there exists a specific subset of cells known as persisters, which are dormant variants that reside deep within the biofilm structure and exhibit resistance to multiple antifungal agents. It is important to note that these persister cells are present in the biofilm community and not within planktonic populations [124]. Rather than being mutants, these cells may be phenotypic variations of the wild type. Studies have demonstrated that the levels of persister cells can range from 0.2 to 9%, with strains isolated from patients suffering chronic carriage displaying higher persister stages compared to strains from patients with transient carriage [115]. Through transcriptional analysis of persister cells, it has been observed that there is diverse regulation of genes involved in the biosynthesis pathways of ergosterol (*ERG1* and *ERG25*) and β-1,6 glucan (*SKN1* and *KRE1*) [125].

3.4 Ergosterols contents and ERG genes expression

Ergosterol is the predominant sterol in the plasma membrane of fungi, which plays a crucial role in the mechanism of action of key antifungal agents like azoles and amphotericin B. These antifungal drugs target lanosterol demethylase, an enzyme involved in the biosynthesis of ergosterol, and hinder the pathway. Studies have indicated that biofilm cells, mainly in the last phases of biofilm creation, had a lower content of ergosterol compared with planktonic cells. Mature biofilm is less dependent on ergosterol for preserving membrane fluidity and the limitation of the effectiveness of antifungals with ergosterol targets. It has been reported that the transcription profile of ergosterol pathway genes (*ERG25*, *ERG11*) is changed, and *ERG11*, which is the main target of antifungal drugs, may be point-mutated or overexpressed in biofilm-producing *Candida albicans* spp. [126].

3.5 Gene overexpression

Increasing the efflux pump is one of the main mechanisms of resistance in azoles, and it reduces drug accumulation in *Candida* cells. Research has shown that in the nonappearance of exposure to antifungals, the expression of *CDR1*, *CDR2*, and *MDR1* is rarely observed. Additionally, the resistance to drugs observed in biofilms may be linked to increased activity of efflux pumps. Studies have demonstrated that in compared to planktonic cells of similar age, *CDR1* and *MDR1* are more commonly transcribed in *C. albicans* biofilms. However, during the mature stage of biofilm formation, the contribution of efflux pumps to antifungal resistance is not significant. It has been reported that efflux pumps play a crucial role in biofilm antifungal resistance during the initial stage of development, as the expression of efflux pump genes is higher after 12 hours of biofilm formation compared to 48 hours. These findings support the theory that efflux pumps may influence the resistance of fungal biofilms to medications, although they are not the sole determining factor. While efflux pumps may contribute to maintaining homeostasis and preventing acute toxicity in complex environments, exposure to azole drugs in clinical settings can increase the expression of efflux pump genes, potentially leading to or contributing to clinical resistance [115, 125–127].

4. Conclusions

Candida spp., a type of pathogenic yeast found in the normal microbiome, can cause infections in individuals with compromised immune systems. Although yeasts are a natural part of the diet and play a role in maintaining the host microbiome, eliminating them completely from the body is neither feasible nor desirable. To treat these infections, various classes of antifungal drugs such as azoles, polyenes, and echinocandins are used. These medications selectively focus on distinct biochemical pathways that are exclusive to yeasts, such as the synthesis of ergosterol, a component that is exclusively present in fungi. The effectiveness of these medications relies on various factors, including the individual's immune system, the severity and location of the infection, and the pharmacokinetics of the drugs. However, there are instances where treatment may fail due to the emergence of drug resistance in *Candida* spp., This comprehensive review provides an in-depth analysis of the molecular mechanisms associated with resistance to antifungal agents. These mechanisms encompass the increased expression of membrane transporters, alterations in the cell wall and ergosterol synthesis, as well as mutations in transcription factors responsible for regulating membrane transporters and ergosterol production. Ongoing research into these mechanisms aims to identify resistant strains, uncover new targets for drug development, and mitigate the occurrence of drug resistance.

Acknowledgements

This work was financially supported through the Pasteur Institute of Iran.

Conflict of interest

The authors have no conflict of interest.

Author details

Simasadat Seyedjavadi, Farahnaz Hatami and Zahra Jahanshiri*
Department of Mycology, Pasteur Institute of Iran, Tehran, Iran

*Address all correspondence to: zjahanshiri@yahoo.com

References

[1] Pfaller MA, Diekema D. Epidemiology of invasive candidiasis: A persistent public health problem. Clinical Microbiology Reviews. 2007;**20**:133-163. DOI: 10.1128/CMR.00029-06

[2] Bhattacharya S, Sae-Tia S, Fries BC. Candidiasis and mechanisms of antifungal resistance. Antibiotics. 2020;**9**:312. DOI: 10.3390/antibiotics9060312

[3] Preventions CfDCa. Drug-Resistant *Candida* Species. Available from: https://www.cdc.gov/drugresistance/pdf/threats-report/*candida*-508.pdf [Accessed: 9 June 2020]

[4] Pfaller M, Neofytos D, Diekema D, Azie N, Meier-Kriesche HU, Quan SP, et al. Epidemiology and outcomes of candidemia in 3648 patients: Data from the Prospective Antifungal Therapy (PATH Alliance®) registry, 2004-2008. Diagnostic Microbiology and Infectious Disease. 2012;**74**:323-331. DOI: 10.1016/j.diagmicrobio.2012.10.003

[5] Kojic EM, Darouiche RO. *Candida* infections of medical devices. Clinical Microbiology Reviews. 2004;**17**:255-267. DOI: 10.1128/CMR.17.2.255-267.2004

[6] Mavor AL, Thewes S, Hube B. Systemic fungal infections caused by *Candida* species: Epidemiology, infection process and virulence attributes. Current Drug Targets. 2005;**6**:863-874. DOI: 10.2174/138945005774912735

[7] Clancy CJ, Nguyen MH. Diagnosing invasive candidiasis. Journal of Clinical Microbiology. 2018;**56**:10-128. DOI: 10.1128/JCM.01909-17

[8] Taddei E, Giovannenze F, Birocchi E, Murri R, Cerolini L, Segala FV, et al. Empiric antifungal therapy for intra-abdominal post-surgical abscesses in non-ICU patients. Antibiotics. 2023;**12**:701. DOI: 10.3390/antibiotics12040701

[9] Ben-Ami R. Treatment of invasive candidiasis: A narrative review. Journal of Fungi. 2018;**4**:97. DOI: 10.3390/jof4030097

[10] Pappas PG, Kauffman CA, Andes DR, Clancy CJ, Marr KA, Ostrosky-Zeichner L, et al. Clinical practice guideline for the management of candidiasis: 2016 update by the Infectious Diseases Society of America. Clinical Infectious Diseases. 2016;**62**:e1-e50. DOI: 10.1093/cid/civ933

[11] Gomez-Lopez A. Antifungal therapeutic drug monitoring: Focus on drugs without a clear recommendation. Clinical Microbiology and Infection. 2020;**26**:1481-1487. DOI: 10.1016/j.cmi.2020.05.037

[12] Carrillo-Munoz AJ, Giusiano G, Ezkurra PA, Quindós G. Antifungal agents: Mode of action in yeast cells. Revista Española de Quimioterapia. 2006;**19**:130-139

[13] Kodedová M, Sychrová H. Changes in the sterol composition of the plasma membrane affect membrane potential, salt tolerance and the activity of multidrug resistance pumps in *Saccharomyces cerevisiae*. PLoS One. 2015;**10**:e0139306. DOI: 10.1371/journal.pone.0139306

[14] Mazu TK, Bricker BA, Flores-Rozas H, Ablordeppey SY. The mechanistic targets of antifungal agents: An overview. Mini Reviews in Medicinal Chemistry. 2016;**16**:555-578. DOI: 10.2174/1389557516666160118112103

[15] Villasmil ML, Barbosa AD, Cunningham JL, Siniossoglou S, Nickels JT Jr. An Erg11 lanosterol 14-α-demethylase-Arv1 complex is required for *Candida albicans* virulence. PLoS One. 2020;**15**:e0235746. DOI: 10.1371/journal.pone.0235746

[16] Delattin N, Cammue BP, Thevissen K. Reactive oxygen species-inducing antifungal agents and their activity against fungal biofilms. Future Medicinal Chemistry. 2014;**6**:77-90. DOI: 10.4155/fmc.13.189

[17] Lamping E, Monk BC, Niimi K, Holmes AR, Tsao S, Tanabe K, et al. Characterization of three classes of membrane proteins involved in fungal azole resistance by functional hyperexpression in *Saccharomyces cerevisiae*. Eukaryotic Cell. 2007;**6**:1150-1165. DOI: 10.1128/EC.00091-07

[18] Coleman JJ, Mylonakis E. Efflux in fungi: la piece de resistance. PLoS Pathogens. 2009;**5**:e1000486. DOI: 10.1371/journal.ppat.1000486

[19] Michealis S, Berkower C. Sequence comparison of yeast ATP-binding cassette proteins. In: Cold Spring Harbor Symposia on Quantitative Biology. Vol. 60. Cold Spring Harbor Laboratory Press; 1995. pp. 291-307. DOI: 10.1101/SQB.1995.060.01.034

[20] Marger MD, Saier MH Jr. A major superfamily of transmembrane facilitators that catalyse uniport, symport and antiport. Trends in Biochemical Sciences. 1993;**18**:13-20. DOI: 10.1016/0968-0004(93)90081-W

[21] Revie NM, Iyer KR, Robbins N, Cowen LE. Antifungal drug resistance: Evolution, mechanisms and impact. Current Opinion in Microbiology. 2018;**45**:70-76. DOI: 10.1016/j.mib.2018.02.005

[22] Robbins N, Caplan T, Cowen LE. Molecular evolution of antifungal drug resistance. Annual Review of Microbiology. 2017;**71**:753-775. DOI: 10.1146/annurev-micro-030117-020345

[23] Tsao S, Rahkhoodaee F, Raymond M. Relative contributions of the *Candida albicans* ABC transporters Cdr1p and Cdr2p to clinical azole resistance. Antimicrobial Agents and Chemotherapy. 2009;**53**:1344-1352. DOI: 10.1128/AAC.00926-08

[24] Coste A, Turner V, Ischer F, Morschhäuser J, Forche A, Selmecki A, et al. A mutation in *Tac1p*, a transcription factor regulating *CDR1* and *CDR2*, is coupled with loss of heterozygosity at chromosome 5 to mediate antifungal resistance in *Candida albicans*. Genetics. 2006;**172**:2139-2156. DOI: 10.1534/genetics.105.054767

[25] White TC. Increased mRNA levels of *ERG16*, *CDR*, and *MDR1* correlate with increases in azole resistance in *Candida albicans* isolates from a patient infected with human immunodeficiency virus. Antimicrobial Agents and Chemotherapy. 1997;**41**:1482-1487. DOI: 10.1128/AAC.41.7.1482

[26] Wirsching S, Michel S, Morschhäuser J. Targeted gene disruption in *Candida albicans* wild-type strains: The role of the *MDR1* gene in fluconazole resistance of clinical *Candida albicans* isolates. Molecular Microbiology. 2000;**36**:856-865. DOI: 10.1046/j.1365-2958.2000.01899.x

[27] Dunkel N, Blaß J, Rogers PD, Morschhäuser J. Mutations in the multi-drug resistance regulator *MRR1*, followed by loss of heterozygosity, are the main cause of *MDR1* overexpression in fluconazole-resistant *Candida albicans* strains. Molecular

Microbiology. 2008;**69**:827-840. DOI: 10.1111/j.1365-2958.2008.06309.x

[28] Morschhäuser J, Barker KS, Liu TT, Blaß-Warmuth J, Homayouni R, Rogers PD. The transcription factor Mrr1p controls expression of the *MDR1* efflux pump and mediates multidrug resistance in *Candida albicans*. PLoS Pathogens. 2007;**3**:e164. DOI: 10.1371/journal.ppat.0030164

[29] Liu Z, Myers LC. *Candida albicans* Swi/Snf and mediator complexes differentially regulate Mrr1-induced *MDR1* expression and fluconazole resistance. Antimicrobial Agents and Chemotherapy. 2017;**61**:10-128. DOI: 10.1128/AAC.01344-17

[30] Marichal P, Koymans L, Willemsens S, Bellens D, Verhasselt P, Luyten W, et al. Contribution of mutations in the cytochrome P450 14α-demethylase (Erg11p, Cyp51p) to azole resistance in *Candida albicans*. Microbiology. 1999;**145**:2701-2713. DOI: 10.1099/00221287-145-10-2701

[31] Xiang MJ, Liu JY, Ni PH, Wang S, Shi C, Wei B, et al. Erg11 mutations associated with azole resistance in clinical isolates of *Candida albicans*. FEMS Yeast Research. 2013;**13**:386-393. DOI: 10.1111/1567-1364.12042

[32] Flowers SA, Colón B, Whaley SG, Schuler MA, Rogers PD. Contribution of clinically derived mutations in *ERG11* to azole resistance in *Candida albicans*. Antimicrobial Agents and Chemotherapy. 2015;**59**:450-460. DOI: 10.1128/AAC.03470-14

[33] Hoot SJ, Smith AR, Brown RP, White TC. An A643V amino acid substitution in Upc2p contributes to azole resistance in well-characterized clinical isolates of *Candida albicans*. Antimicrobial Agents and Chemotherapy. 2011;**55**:940-942. DOI: 10.1128/AAC.00995-10

[34] Heilmann CJ, Schneider S, Barker KS, Rogers PD, Morschhäuser J. An A643T mutation in the transcription factor Upc2p causes constitutive *ERG11* upregulation and increased fluconazole resistance in *Candida albicans*. Antimicrobial Agents and Chemotherapy. 2010;**54**:353-359. DOI: 10.1128/AAC.01102-09

[35] Cowen LE, Steinbach WJ. Stress, drugs, and evolution: The role of cellular signaling in fungal drug resistance. Eukaryotic Cell. 2008;**7**:747-764. DOI: 10.1128/EC.00041-08

[36] Kelly SL, Lamb DC, Kelly DE, Manning NJ, Loeffler J, Hebart H, et al. Resistance to fluconazole and cross-resistance to amphotericin B in *Candida albicans* from AIDS patients caused by defective sterol Δ5, 6-desaturation. FEBS Letters. 1997;**400**:80-82. DOI: 10.1016/S0014-5793(96)01360-9

[37] Morio F, Pagniez F, Lacroix C, Miegeville M, Le Pape P. Amino acid substitutions in the *Candida albicans* sterol Δ5, 6-desaturase (Erg3p) confer azole resistance: Characterization of two novel mutants with impaired virulence. Journal of Antimicrobial Chemotherapy. 2012;**67**:2131-2138. DOI: 10.1093/jac/dks186

[38] Cowen LE. The fungal Achilles' heel: Targeting Hsp90 to cripple fungal pathogens. Current Opinion in Microbiology. 2013;**16**:377-384. DOI: 10.1016/j.mib.2013.03.005

[39] Taipale M, Krykbaeva I, Koeva M, Kayatekin C, Westover KD, Karras GI, et al. Quantitative analysis of HSP90-client interactions reveals principles of substrate recognition. Cell. 2012;**150**:987-1001. DOI: 10.1016/j.cell.2012.06.047

[40] Jarosz DF, Taipale M, Lindquist S. Protein homeostasis and the phenotypic manifestation of genetic diversity: Principles and mechanisms. Annual Review of Genetics. 2010;**44**:189-216. DOI: 10.1146/annurev.genet.40.110405.090412

[41] Cowen LE, Lindquist S. Hsp90 potentiates the rapid evolution of new traits: Drug resistance in diverse fungi. Science. 2005;**309**:2185-2189. DOI: 10.1126/science.1118370

[42] Singh SD, Robbins N, Zaas AK, Schell WA, Perfect JR, Cowen LE. Hsp90 governs echinocandin resistance in the pathogenic yeast *Candida albicans* via calcineurin. PLoS Pathogens. 2009;**5**:e1000532. DOI: 10.1371/journal.ppat.1000532

[43] Cruz MC, Goldstein AL, Blankenship JR, Del Poeta M, Davis D, Cardenas ME, et al. Calcineurin is essential for survival during membrane stress in *Candida albicans*. The EMBO Journal. 2002;**21**:546-559. DOI: 10.1093/emboj/21.4.546

[44] LaFayette SL, Collins C, Zaas AK, Schell WA, Betancourt-Quiroz M, Gunatilaka AL, et al. PKC signaling regulates drug resistance of the fungal pathogen *Candida albicans* via circuitry comprised of Mkc1, calcineurin, and Hsp90. PLoS Pathogens. 2010;**6**:e1001069. DOI: 10.1371/journal.ppat.1001069

[45] Robbins N, Collins C, Morhayim J, Cowen LE. Metabolic control of antifungal drug resistance. Fungal Genetics and Biology. 2010;**47**:81-93. DOI: 10.1016/j.fgb.2009.07.004

[46] Robbins N, Wright GD, Cowen LE. Antifungal drugs: The current armamentarium and development of new agents. Microbiology Spectrum. 2016;**4**:4-5. DOI: 10.1128/microbiolspec.FUNK-0002-2016

[47] Li X, Robbins N, O'Meara TR, Cowen LE. Extensive functional redundancy in the regulation of *C andida albicans* drug resistance and morphogenesis by lysine deacetylases H os2, H da1, R pd3 and R pd31. Molecular Microbiology. 2017;**103**:635-656. DOI: 10.1111/mmi.13578

[48] Selmecki A, Forche A, Berman J. Genomic plasticity of the human fungal pathogen *Candida albicans*. Eukaryotic Cell. 2010;**9**:991-1008. DOI: 10.1128/EC.00060-10

[49] Chen G, Rubinstein B, Li R. Whole chromosome aneuploidy: Big mutations drive adaptation by phenotypic leap. BioEssays. 2012;**34**:893-900. DOI: 10.1002/bies.201200069

[50] Harrison BD, Hashemi J, Bibi M, Pulver R, Bavli D, Nahmias Y, et al. A tetraploid intermediate precedes aneuploid formation in yeasts exposed to fluconazole. PLoS Biology. 2014;**12**:e1001815. DOI: 10.1371/journal.pbio.1001815

[51] Selmecki A, Gerami-Nejad M, Paulson C, Forche A, Berman J. An isochromosome confers drug resistance in vivo by amplification of two genes, ERG11 and TAC1. Molecular Microbiology. 2008;**68**:624-641. DOI: 10.1111/j.1365-2958.2008.06176.x

[52] Anderson MZ, Saha A, Haseeb A, Bennett RJ. A chromosome 4 trisomy contributes to increased fluconazole resistance in a clinical isolate of *Candida albicans*. Microbiology. 2017;**163**:856. DOI: 10.1099/mic.0.000478

[53] Hill JA, Ammar R, Torti D, Nislow C, Cowen LE. Genetic and genomic architecture of the

evolution of resistance to antifungal drug combinations. PLoS Genetics. 2013;**9**:e1003390. DOI: 10.1371/journal.pgen.1003390

[54] Forche A, Abbey D, Pisithkul T, Weinzierl MA, Ringstrom T, Bruck D, et al. Stress alters rates and types of loss of heterozygosity in *Candida albicans*. MBio. 2011;**2**:10-128. DOI: 10.1128/mBio.00129-11

[55] Ferrari S, Sanguinetti M, Torelli R, Posteraro B, Sanglard D. Contribution of *CgPDR1*-regulated genes in enhanced virulence of azole-resistant *Candida glabrata*. PLoS One. 2011;**6**:e17589. DOI: 10.1371/journal.pone.0017589

[56] Borst A, Raimer MT, Warnock DW, Morrison CJ, Arthington-Skaggs BA. Rapid acquisition of stable azole resistance by *Candida glabrata* isolates obtained before the clinical introduction of fluconazole. Antimicrobial Agents and Chemotherapy. 2005;**49**:783-787. DOI: 10.1128/AAC.49.2.783-787.2005

[57] Sanglard D, Ischer F, Bille J. Role of ATP-binding-cassette transporter genes in high-frequency acquisition of resistance to azole antifungals in *Candida glabrata*. Antimicrobial Agents and Chemotherapy. 2001;**45**:1174-1183. DOI: 10.1128/AAC.45.4.1174-1183.2001

[58] Blankenship JR, Mitchell AP. How to build a biofilm: A fungal perspective. Current Opinion in Microbiology. 2006;**9**:588-594. DOI: 10.1016/j.mib.2006.10.003

[59] Douglas LJ. *Candida* biofilms and their role in infection. Trends in Microbiology. 2003;**11**:30-36. DOI: 10.1016/S0966-842X(02)00002-1

[60] Mayer FL, Wilson D, Hube B. *Candida albicans* pathogenicity mechanisms. Virulence. 2013;**4**:119-128. DOI: 10.4161/viru.22913

[61] Ramage G, Bachmann S, Patterson TF, Wickes BL, López-Ribot JL. Investigation of multidrug efflux pumps in relation to fluconazole resistance in *Candida albicans* biofilms. Journal of Antimicrobial Chemotherapy. 2002;**49**:973-980. DOI: 10.1093/jac/dkf049

[62] Nett JE, Crawford K, Marchillo K, Andes DR. Role of Fks1p and matrix glucan in *Candida albicans* biofilm resistance to an echinocandin, pyrimidine, and polyene. Antimicrobial Agents and Chemotherapy. 2010;**54**:3505-3508. DOI: 10.1128/AAC.00227-10

[63] Efimova SS, Schagina LV, Ostroumova OS. Investigation of channel-forming activity of polyene macrolide antibiotics in planar lipid bilayers in the presence of dipole modifiers. Acta Naturae (англоязычная версия). 2014;**6**:67-79. DOI: 10.32607/20758251-2014-6-4-67-79

[64] Hamill RJ. Amphotericin B formulations: A comparative review of efficacy and toxicity. Drugs. 2013;**73**:919-934. DOI: 10.1007/s40265-013-0069-4

[65] Vogelsinger H, Weiler S, Djanani A, Kountchev J, Bellmann-Weiler R, Wiedermann CJ, et al. Amphotericin B tissue distribution in autopsy material after treatment with liposomal amphotericin B and amphotericin B colloidal dispersion. Journal of Antimicrobial Chemotherapy. 2006;**57**:1153-1160. DOI: 10.1093/jac/dkl141

[66] Odds FC, Brown AJP, Gow NAR. Antifungal agents: Mechanisms of action. Trends in Microbiology. 2003;**11**:272-279. DOI: 10.1016/s0966-842x(03)00117-3

[67] Kumar R, Shukla PK. Amphotericin B resistance leads to enhanced proteinase and phospholipase activity and reduced germ tube formation in *Candida albicans*. Fungal Biology. 2010;**114**:189-197. DOI: 10.1016/j.funbio.2009.12.003

[68] Athar MA, Winner HI. The development of resistance by *Candida* species to polyene antibiotics in vitro. Journal of Medical Microbiology. 1971;**4**:505-517. DOI: 10.1099/00222615-4-4-505

[69] Carolus H, Pierson S, Lagrou K, Van Dijck P. Amphotericin B and other polyenes—Discovery, clinical use, mode of action and drug resistance. Journal of Fungi. 2020;**6**:321. DOI: 10.3390/jof6040321

[70] Kamiński DM. Recent progress in the study of the interactions of amphotericin B with cholesterol and ergosterol in lipid environments. European Biophysics Journal. 2014;**43**:453-467. DOI: 10.1007/s00249-014-0983-8

[71] Kristanc L, Božič B, Jokhadar ŠZ, Dolenc MS, Gomišček G. The pore-forming action of polyenes: From model membranes to living organisms. Biochimica et Biophysica Acta (BBA)-Biomembranes. 2019;**1861**:418-430. DOI: 10.1016/j.bbamem.2018.11.006

[72] Matsuoka S, Ikeuchi H, Matsumori N, Murata M. Dominant formation of a single-length channel by amphotericin B in dimyristoylphosphatidylcholine membrane evidenced by 13C–31P rotational echo double resonance. Biochemistry. 2005;**44**:704-770. DOI: 10.1021/bi049001k

[73] Guo X, Zhang J, Li X, Xiao E, Lange JD, Rienstra CM, et al. Sterol sponge mechanism is conserved for glycosylated polyene macrolides. ACS Central Science. 2021;**7**:781-791. DOI: 10.1021/acscentsci.1c00148

[74] Anderson TM, Clay MC, Cioffi AG, |Diaz KA, Hisao GS, Tuttle MD, et al. Amphotericin forms an extramembranous and fungicidal sterol sponge. Nature Chemical Biology. 2014;**10**:400-406. DOI: 10.1038/nchembio.1496

[75] McCarthy M, O'Shaughnessy EM, Walsh TJ. Amphotericin B: Polyene resistance mechanisms. Antimicrobial Drug Resistance. 2017;**1**:387-395. DOI: 10.1007/978-3-319-46718-4_26

[76] Thannickal VJ, Fanburg BL. Reactive oxygen species in cell signaling. American Journal of Physiology-lung Cellular and Molecular Physiology. 2000;**279**:L1005-L1028. DOI: 10.1152/ajplung.2000.279.6.L1005

[77] Farber JL. Mechanisms of cell injury by activated oxygen species. Enviromental Health Perspectives. 1994;**102**:S17-S24. DOI: 10.1289/ehp.94102s1017

[78] Andrews FA, Sarosi GA, Beggs WH. Enhancement of amphotericin B activity by a series of compounds related to phenolic antioxidants. Journal of Antimicrobial Chemotherapy. 1979;**5**:173-177. DOI: 10.1093/jac/5.2.173

[79] Blum G, Hörtnagl C, Jukic E. New insight into amphotericin B resistance in Aspergillus terreus. Antimicrobial Agents and Chemotherapy. 2013;**57**:1583-1588. DOI: 10.1128/AAC.01283-12

[80] Lockhart SR, Iqbal N, Cleveland AA, Farley MM, Harrison LH, Bolden CB, et al. Species identification and antifungal susceptibility testing of *Candida* bloodstream isolates from population-based surveillance studies in two U.S. cities from 2008 to 2011. Journal of Clinical Microbiology. 2012;**50**:3435-3442. DOI: 10.1128/JCM.01283-12

[81] Nagoba BS, Shaikh N, Jahagirdar V, Kothadia S. Antifungal drug resistance in *Candida* species. European Journal of General Medicine. 2013;**10**:254-258

[82] Branco J, Miranda IM, Rodrigues AG. *Candida parapsilosis* virulence and antifungal resistance mechanisms: A comprehensive review of key determinants. Journal of Fungi. 2023;**9**:80. DOI: 10.3390/jof9010080

[83] Lee Y, Puumala E, Robbins N, Cowen LE. Antifungal drug resistance: Molecular mechanisms *in Candida albicans* and beyond. Chemical Reviews. 2020;**121**:3390-3411. DOI: 10.1021/acs.chemrev.0c00199

[84] Anderson JB, Sirjusingh C, Syed N. Gene expression and evolution of antifungal drug resistance. Antimicrobial Agents and Chemotherapy. 2009;**53**:1931-1936. DOI: 10.1128/AAC.01315-08

[85] Vincent BM, Lancaster AK, Scherz-Shouval R, Whitesell L, Lindquist S. Fitness trade-offs restrict the evolution of resistance to Amphotericin B. PLoS Biology. 2013;**11**:e1001692. DOI: 10.1371/journal.pbio.1001692

[86] Seo K, Akiyoshi H, Ohnishi Y. Alteration of cell wall composition leads to amphotericin B resistance in *Aspergillus flavus*. Microbiology and Immunology. 1999;**43**:1017-1025. DOI: 10.1111/j.1348-0421.1999.tb01231.x

[87] Popolo L, Gualtieri T, Ragni E. The yeast cell-wall salvage pathway. Sabouraudia. 2001;**39**:111-121. DOI: 10.1080/744118881

[88] Perlin DS. Current perspectives on echinocandin class drugs. Future Microbiology. 2011;**6**:441-457. DOI: 10.2217/fmb.11.19

[89] Szymanskia M, Chmielewskab S, Czyzewskaa U, Malinowskac M, Tylickia A. Echinocandins – Structure, mechanism of action and use in antifungal therapy. Journal of Enzyme Inhibition and Medical chemistry. 2022;**37**:876-894. DOI: 10.1080/14756366.2022.2050224

[90] Cappelletty D, Eiselstein-McKitrick K. The echinocandins. Pharmacotherapy. 2007;**27**:369-388. DOI: 10.1592/phco.27.3.369

[91] Perlin DS. Echinocandin resistance in *Candida*. Clinical Infectious Diseases. 2015;**61**:612-617. DOI: 10.1093/cid/civ791

[92] Pappas PG, Kauman CA, Andes DR, Clancy CJ, Marr KA, Ostrosky-Zeichner L, et al. Executive summary: Clinical practice guideline for the management of candidiasis: 2016 update by the Infectious Diseases Society of America. Clinical Infection Disease. 2016;**62**:409-417. DOI: 10.1093/cid/civ1194

[93] Coste AT, Kritikos A, Li J, Khanna N, Goldenberger D, Garzoni C, et al. Emerging echinocandin-resistant *Candida albicans* and *glabrata* in Switzerland. Infection. 2020;**48**:761-766. DOI: 10.1007/s15010-020-01475-8

[94] Healey KR, Perlin DS. Fungal resistance to echinocandins and the MDR phenomenon in *Candida glabrata*. Journal of Fungi. 2018;**4**:105-118. DOI: 10.3390/jof4030105

[95] Shields RK, Nguyen MH, Press EG, Cumbie R, Driscoll E, Pasculle AW. Rate of FKS mutations among consecutive *candida* isolates causing bloodstream infection. Antimicrobial Agents and Chemotherapy. 2015;**59**:7465-7470. DOI: 10.1128/AAC.01973 -15

[96] Garcia-Effron G, Lee S, Park S, Cleary JD, Perlin DS. Effect of *Candida*

glabrata FKS1 and *FKS2* mutations on echinocandin sensitivity and kinetics of 1,3-beta-D-glucan synthase: Implication for the existing susceptibility breakpoint. Antimicrobial Agents and Chemotherapy. 2009;**53**:3690-3699. DOI: 10.1128/AAC.00443-09

[97] Hashimoto S. Micafungin: A sulfated echinocandin. Journal of Antibiotics. 2009;**62**:27-35. DOI: 10.1038/ja.2008.3

[98] Review on current status of echinocandins use. Antiiotics. 2020;**9**:227. DOI: 10.3390/antibiotics9050227

[99] Arendrup MC, Jørgensen KM, Hare RK, Cuenca-Estrella M, Zaragoza O. EUCAST reference testing of Rezafungin susceptibility and impact of choice of plastic plates. Antimicrobial Agents and Chemotherapy. 2019;**63**:e00659-e00619

[100] Vermes A, Guchelaar HJ, Dankert J. Flucytosine: A review of its pharmacology, clinical indications, pharmacokinetics, toxicity and drug interactions. Journal of Antimicrobial Chemotherapy. 2000;**1**(46):171-179. DOI: 10.1093/jac/46.2.171

[101] Perfect JR, Dismukes WE, Dromer F, Goldman DL, Graybill JR, Hamill RJ, et al. Clinical practice guidelines for the management of cryptococcal disease: 2010 update by the Infectious Diseases Society of America. Clinical Infectious Diseases. 2010;**1**(50):291-322. DOI: 10.1086/649858

[102] Whelan WL. The genetic basis of resistance to 5-fluorocytosine *in Candida* species and *Cryptococcus neoformans*. CRC Critical Reviews in Microbiology. 1987;**1**(15):45-56. DOI: 10.3109/10408418709104447

[103] Cowen LE, Sanglard D, Howard SJ, Rogers PD, Perlin DS. Mechanisms of antifungal drug resistance. Cold Spring Harbor Perspectives in Medicine. 2015;**5**(7):a019752. DOI: 10.1101/cshperspect.a019752

[104] Delma FZ, Al-Hatmi AM, Brüggemann RJ, Melchers WJ, de Hoog S, Verweij PE, et al. Molecular mechanisms of 5-fluorocytosine resistance in yeasts and filamentous fungi. Journal of Fungi. 2021;**27**(7):909. DOI: 10.3390/jof7110909

[105] Pfaller MA, Messer SA, Boyken L, Huynh H, Hollis RJ, Diekema DJ. In vitro activities of 5-fluorocytosine against 8,803 clinical isolates of *Candida* spp.: Global assessment of primary resistance using National Committee for Clinical Laboratory Standards susceptibility testing methods. Antimicrobial Agents and chemotherapy. 2002;**46**:3518-3521. DOI: 10.1128/AAC.46.11.3518-3521.2002

[106] Cuenca-Estrella MT, Diaz-Guerra TM, Mellado E, Rodriguez-Tudela JL. Flucytosine primary resistance in *Candida* species and *Cryptococcus neoformans*. European Journal of Clinical Microbiology and Infectious Diseases. 2001;**20**:276-279. DOI: 10.1007/PL00011265

[107] Barchiesi F, Arzeni D, Caselli F, Scalise G. Primary resistance to flucytosine among clinical isolates of *Candida* spp. Journal of Antimicrobial Chemotherapy. 2000;**1**(45):408-409. DOI: 10.1093/jac/45.3.408

[108] Chapeland-Leclerc F, Bouchoux J, Goumar A, Chastin C, Villard J, Noël T. Inactivation of the FCY2 gene encoding purine-cytosine permease promotes cross-resistance to flucytosine and fluconazole in *Candida lusitaniae*. Antimicrobial Agents and Chemotherapy. 2005;**49**:3101-3108. DOI: 10.1128/AAC.49.8.3101-3108

[109] Dodgson AR, Dodgson KJ, Pujol C, Pfaller MA, Soll DR. Clade-specific

flucytosine resistance is due to a single nucleotide change in the FUR1 gene of *Candida albicans*. Antimicrobial Agents and Chemotherapy. 2004;**48**:2223-2227. DOI: 10.1128/AAC.48.6.2223-2227.2004

[110] Taff HT, Mitchell KF, Edward JA, Andes DR. Mechanisms of *Candida* biofilm drug resistance. Future Microbiology. 2013;**8**:1325-1337. DOI: 10.2217/fmb.13.101

[111] Kolter R, Greenberg EP. Microbial sciences: The superficial life of microbes. Nature. 2006;**441**:300-302. DOI: 10.1038/441300a

[112] Gulati M, Nobile CJ. *Candida albicans* biofilms: Development, regulation, and molecular mechanisms. Microbes Infection. 2016;**18**:310-321. DOI: 10.1016/j.micinf.2016.01.002

[113] Chandra J, Mukherjee P. *Candida* biofilms: Development, architecture, and resistance. Microbiology Spectrum. 2015;**3**:157-176. DOI: 10.1128/microbiolspec. MB-0020-2015

[114] Nett JE, Andes DR. Contributions of the biofilm matrix to *Candida* pathogenesis. Journal of Fungi. 2020;**6**:E21. DOI: 10.3390/jof6010021

[115] Silva S, Rodrigues CF, Araújo D, Rodrigues ME, Henriques M. Candida species biofilms' antifungal resistance. Journal of Fungi. 2017;**3**(1):8. DOI: 10.3390/jof3010008

[116] Rajendran R, Sherry L, Nile CJ, Sherriff A, Johnson EM, Hanson MF, et al. Biofilm formation is a risk factor for mortality in patients with *Candida albicans* bloodstream infection- Scotland, 2012-2013. Clinical Microbiology Infection. 2016;**22**:87-93. DOI: 10.1016/j.cmi.2015.09.018

[117] Dominguez E, Zarnowski R, Sanchez H, Covelli AS, Westler WM, Azadi P, et al. Conservation and divergence in the *Candida* species biofilm matrix mannanglucan complex structure, function, and genetic control. MBio. 2018;**9**:e00451-e00418. DOI: 10.1128/mBio.00451-18

[118] Seneviratne CJ, Jin L, Samaranayake LP. Biofilm lifestyle of *Candida*: A mini review. Oral Disease. 2008;**14**:582-590. DOI: 10.1111/j.1601-0825.2007.01424.x

[119] Donlan RM, Costerton JW. Biofilms: Survival mechanisms of clinically relevant microorganisms. Clinical Microbiology Review. 2002;**15**:167-193. DOI: 10.1128/CMR.15.2.167-193.2002

[120] Silva S, Negri M, Henriques M, Oliveira R, Williams D, Azeredo J. *Candida glabrata*, *Candida parapsilosis* and *Candida tropicalis*: Biology, epidemiology, pathogenicity and antifungal resistance. FEMS Microbiology Review. 2012;**36**:288-205. DOI: 10.1111/j.1574-6976.2011.00278.x

[121] Martins M, Henriques M, Lopez-Ribot JL, Oliveira R. Addition of DNase improves the in vitro activity of antifungal drugs against *Candida albicans* biofilms. Mycoses. 2012;**55**:80-85. DOI: 10.1111/j.1439-0507.2011.02047.x

[122] Knot PD, Suci PA, Miller RL, Nelson RD, Tyler BJ. A small subpopulation of blastospores in *Candida albicans* biofilms exhibit resistance to amphotericin B associated with differential regulation of ergosterol and −1,6-glucan pathway genes. Antimicrobial Agents and Chemotherapy. 2006;**50**:3708-3716. DOI: 10.1128/AAC.00997-06

[123] Nobile CJ, Nett JE, Hernday AD, Homann OR, Deneault J-S,

Nantel A, et al. Biofilm matrix regulation by *Candida albicans Zap1*. PLoS Biology. 2009;7:e1000133. DOI: 10.1371/journal.pbio.1000133

[124] LaFleur MD, Kumamoto CA, Lewis K. *Candida albicans* biofilms produce antifungal-tolerant persister cells. Antimicrobial Agents and Chemotherapy. 2006;**50**:3839-3846. DOI: 10.1128/AAC.00684-06

[125] Mukherjee PK, Chandra J, Kuhn DM, Ghannoum MA. Mechanism of fluconazole resistance in *Candida albicans* biofilms: Phase-specific role of efflux pumps and membrane sterols. Infection and Immunology. 2003;**71**:4333-4340. DOI: 10.1128/IAI.71.8.4333-4340.2003

[126] Schubert S, Barker KS, Znaidi S, Schneider S, Dierolf F, Dunkel N, et al. Regulation of efflux pump expression and drug resistance by the transcription factors *Mrr1*, *Upc2*, and *Cap1* in *Candida albicans*. Antimicrobial Agents and Chemotherapy. 2011;**55**:2212-2223. DOI: 10.1128/AAC.01343-10

[127] Ramage G, Rajendran R, Sherry L, Williams C. Fungal biofilm resistance. International Journal of Microbiology. 2012;**2012**(1):528521. DOI: 10.1155/2012/528521

Chapter 6

Nanomaterial against *Candida albicans*

Sobhan Mortazavi-Derazkola, Seyedeh Masoumeh Ghoreishi, Pouria Mohammadparast-Tabas, Hamed Aramjoo and Azar Bazrgaran

Abstract

In recent years, there has been a significant increase in the resistance of microorganisms to common treatments, among which *Candida albicans* (*C. albicans*) is no exception. Due to the eukaryotic nature of fungi, antifungal drugs have less variety than antibiotics. Additionally, the formation of biofilm by fungi serves as a physical barrier, reducing the effectiveness of antifungal drugs. Consequently, several studies are currently underway to explore new treatments to prevent *C. albicans* infection. Nanotechnology in medicine has rapidly advanced in recent years, demonstrating satisfactory results in various fields. Nanomaterials can function as antifungal drugs and act as carriers and protectors of antifungal agents. These unique properties of nanomaterials position them as promising treatments for eliminating infections caused by *C. albicans*. In the following sections, we will discuss some recent developments in utilizing nanomaterials for the treatment of *C. albicans* infections.

Keywords: nanomaterials, metal nanoparticle, nanocomplex, mesoporous silica nanoparticle, liposomal nanoparticle, polymeric nanoparticle

1. Introduction

Candidiasis represents an opportunistic fungal infection caused by Candida spp., affecting diverse anatomical sites, including the skin, oral cavity, gastrointestinal tract, and reproductive tract. Systemic candidiasis poses a life-threatening risk and is estimated to occur globally at approximately four million cases annually [1, 2].

This infection particularly impacts immunocompromised individuals, such as transplant recipients, those in intensive care, post-surgery patients, individuals with cancer, and those living with HIV. It exerts significant economic burden due to the elevated expenses associated with medication and prolonged hospital stays [3, 4]. *Candida albicans* (*C. albicans*) stands out as the most virulent yeast species, predominantly responsible for both superficial and systemic infections [5].

Numerous factors and mechanisms contribute to the pathogenicity of *C. albicans*. These encompass molecules facilitating adhesion to and invasion of host cells, the secretion of hydrolases, the transition from yeast to hyphae, contact sensing and thigmotropism, biofilm formation, phenotypic switching, and various fitness attributes [6]. *C. albicans* exhibits a form of adaptability termed morphogenesis, entailing a transition from a yeast form to a hyphal form. This morphological alteration enables *C. albicans* to effectively penetrate mucous membranes, invade tissues, and enter the bloodstream, thereby increasing the risk of tissue damage. Moreover, morphogenesis aids *C. albicans* in evading macrophage phagocytosis. Another virulent trait of *C. albicans* is its ability to form biofilms on both abiotic and biotic surfaces [7].

The escalation in Candida infections is attributed to its increasing resistance to antifungal agents. Various antifungal medications, predominantly azoles, are utilized for treating candidiasis. Depending on the infection type and location, polyenes, echinocandins, allylamines, and nucleoside analogs are also employed. However, the effectiveness of these drugs is waning due to Candida's adeptness at adapting and surviving, even in the presence of high concentrations of these antifungal agents. Fungi share the same eukaryotic structure and metabolism as their hosts, complicating treatment. Consequently, there is an urgent and unavoidable demand for antifungals featuring novel antimicrobial mechanisms [8, 9].

Fortunately, nanotechnology provides a promising avenue for developing new antimicrobial agents. Nanoparticles (NPs), composed of lipids [10], polymers [11], or metals [12], typically range in size from 1 to 100 nm. Materials at these dimensions exhibit unique characteristics absent in bulk materials [13]. NPs offer several advantages over traditional drugs [14], including increased targeting accuracy at infection sites, larger surface area, reduced toxic effects and side effects, and lower likelihood of inducing resistance [15]. Additionally, NPs can protect the drug from degradation [16], enhance drug stability [17], and facilitate drug entry into *C. albicans* [18]. The attributes conferred by NPs have enhanced the efficacy of existing antifungal drugs or produced substances with antifungal properties, showing promising results. This chapter of the book explores the anti-*C. albicans* activity of various NPs, encompassing metal NPs and nanocomplexes, mesoporous silica NPs, liposomes, and polymers, considering their diverse applications.

2. Metal NPs

The emergence of NPs has opened up novel avenues for their application as nano-drugs. Numerous metals display antibacterial and antifungal properties, and NPs derived from these metals also exhibit these characteristics [19]. In metal NPs, the reduction in volume results in an increase in the surface-to-volume ratio. This elevation in ratio enhances the interaction of bacteria and fungi with NPs, markedly enhancing their antibacterial and antifungal properties compared to the bulk state [20]. Metal NPs offer advantages such as facile decomposition, UV optical activity, catalytic activity, chemical stability, low toxicity, and adjustable size, garnering significant attention from researchers [21].

Controlling the synthesis process of NPs can impact their size, shape, charge, hydrophobicity, and porosity. These parameters, in turn, influence stability, biocompatibility, circulation time in the bloodstream, treatment targeting, and the cellular entry of NPs [22]. Generally, two methods exist for NPs synthesis: the top-down method and the bottom-up method. The top-down method involves the physical synthesis of NPs, utilizing techniques such as sputtering, chemical etching, ball milling, sonication, laser ablation, and electro-explosion. While this method necessitates sophisticated tools and equipment and is time-consuming and expensive, it facilitates the transformation of materials from bulk to NPs [23]. In contrast, the bottom-up method entails the chemical or biological synthesis of NPs. Accumulation of atoms gives rise to NPs in techniques such as laser pyrolysis, sol-gel, spinning, spray pyrolysis, atomic condensation, and chemical vapor deposition (**Figure 1**). However, chemical methods of NP synthesis present drawbacks such as environmental toxicity, low efficiency, high energy consumption, and toxicity when applied for biological purposes [24]. The biological method involves the synthesis of NPs using plant extracts (leaf, root, fruit, flower, or seed extracts) or microorganisms (bacteria, fungi, or algae). Compared to chemical and physical methods, the biological approach offers greater stability, efficiency, lower cost, and absence of biological toxicity, rendering it more favorable for NP synthesis [25].

Among metal NPs, gold (Au) NPs have garnered considerable attention due to their biochemical, sensory, optical, and electronic properties, as well as their biocompatibility, low toxicity, ease of synthesis, and adjustable size [26]. Additionally, Au NPs are among the NPs approved by the FDA, further promoting their utilization [27]. Au NPs can also conjugate with biological molecules such as peptides, enzymes, and DNA, enhancing stability and reducing the side effects of drugs [28, 29]. Various studies have investigated the effects of Au NPs on *C. albicans* fungus based on their characteristics. The size of the NPs is the most critical factor influencing the anti-Candida activity of Au NPs [30]. Au NPs have demonstrated the ability to inhibit the aspartyl proteinase 2 enzyme in a dose- and time-dependent manner [31]. Moreover, Au NPs have exhibited low cytotoxicity against fibroblast cell lines and blood cells [32]. In a study by Salehi et al., Au NPs synthesized together with the drug caspofungin showed enhanced anti-candida effects compared to caspofungin alone [33]. Au NPs can also be synthesized through green methods. In Kareem et al.'s study, Au NPs synthesized using olive leaf extract displayed high efficacy in killing *C. albicans* fungus and effectively treating skin candidiasis in mice [34]. Based on these findings, Au NPs possess significant therapeutic potential for combating *C. albicans* fungus.

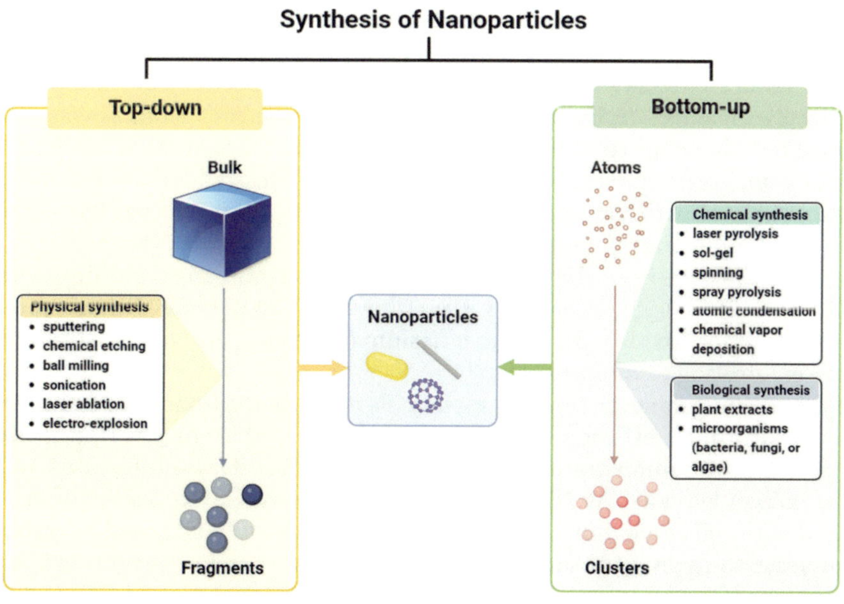

Figure 1.
Different methods of nanoparticle synthesis.

Another group of metal NPs, known as one of the most crucial antimicrobial NPs, are silver (Ag) NPs [35]. Ag NPs have been extensively studied in biomedicine for anticancer drugs, vaccines, and drug delivery systems [36]. Ag NPs exhibit potent antimicrobial properties against various microbes, including drug-resistant strains [37]. They can be easily synthesized, and numerous studies have demonstrated their anti-Candida effects [38]. Ag NPs have been shown to eradicate fluconazole-resistant *C. albicans* clinical isolates [39]. Additionally, Ag NPs conjugated with amphotericin B displayed enhanced anti-*C. albicans* activity compared to amphotericin B and Ag NPs alone [16]. Utilizing Ag NPs as carriers of antifungal drugs can reduce drug concentration and toxicity while enhancing treatment effectiveness. In Jia et al.'s study, the combination of Ag NPs with fluconazole effectively eradicated fluconazole-resistant *C. albicans* and improved treatment efficacy in infected mice [40]. Due to the toxicity associated with Ag NPs, the green synthesis method is predominantly employed for their synthesis. Various studies have synthesized Ag NPs using different plant extracts, such as *Lotus lalambensis* [13], *Zingiber officinale* [41], and *Carum carvi* [42], demonstrating their efficacy in destroying *C. albicans* fungus. Moreover, Ag NPs have shown high anti-biofilm activity [43].

Zinc-containing NPs, such as zinc oxide (ZnO) NPs, are noteworthy for their antifungal and antimicrobial properties, attributed to their low solubility, biocompatibility, and low toxicity [44]. Research has demonstrated that ZnO NPs, either alone or in combination with drugs like fluconazole [45] and nystatin [46], exhibit significant antifungal activity. Moreover, ZnO NPs synthesized through green methods have shown substantial anti-Candida activity [47]. In the study by Pillai et al., various plant extracts were utilized, resulting in different levels of antifungal activity in ZnO NPs [48].

Iron oxide NPs are recognized for their high chemical stability, cost-effectiveness, significant surface-to-volume and surface-to-weight ratios, and superparamagnetic properties. These characteristics make them suitable for biomedical applications and drug delivery systems [49]. The antifungal efficacy of iron oxide NPs against species like *C. albicans* has been established in several studies [50, 51]. Recent advancements in modifying their size, shape, and surface coating have enhanced their biocompatibility and reduced toxicity [52]. In a study by Balabathula et al., iron oxide NPs were synthesized with amphotericin B. Enhanced activity against *C. albicans* was observed when used together compared to amphotericin B alone. Transmission Electron Microscopy images in this study indicated that the synthesized NPs penetrated *C. albicans* cells [18]. Furthermore, green synthesis of iron oxide NPs has been explored, with studies demonstrating their high efficacy against *C. albicans* [53, 54].

Selenium NPs have been shown to bind to and penetrate fungal biofilms, exhibiting antifungal effects [55]. Other NPs, including titanium dioxide [56], zirconium dioxide [57], copper oxide [58], and magnesium oxide [59], also demonstrate capabilities in eradicating *C. albicans* cells.

The overarching concern in using metal NPs is balancing toxicity reduction with maximized antifungal efficacy, often achieved through different covering agents.

Metal NPs have demonstrated efficacy in reducing *C. albicans* infections. In a study by Halbandge et al., Ag NPs were found to decrease the expression of genes associated with cell elongation (ECE1), hyphae induction (TEC1), and negative regulation of yeast-to-hyphae transition (TUP1 and RFG1), thereby preventing *C. albicans* infections [60]. Additionally, Muthamil et al. discovered that Ag NPs not only inhibit the yeast-to-hyphae transition but also reduce exopolysaccharide synthesis in

C. albicans. These NPs also decrease the secretion of aspartyl proteinase, a key factor in fungal pathogenicity [61]. Ag NPs have further been observed to prevent the formation of germ tubes and biofilms in *C. albicans* [62].

The effectiveness of NPs is directly correlated with the amount and nature of ions they release [63]. The mechanism by which metal NPs eradicate *C. albicans* involves initial adherence to the fungal cell membrane. These NPs disrupt the function of proteins on the fungal cell wall, particularly beta-glucan synthase, whose disruption impairs cell wall synthesis [64]. Subsequently, the NPs penetrate the fungal cell, releasing metal ions internally. The presence of NPs on the cell membrane and the resulting ion release disturb cell wall integrity, membrane transport, and membrane fluidity [65]. Transmission electron microscopy studies have illustrated that metal NPs can disrupt the cell wall and membrane of *C. albicans*, resulting in the leakage of intracellular contents [66]. Radhakrishnan et al. observed that Ag NPs affect the surface morphology, membrane microenvironment, fluidity, and composition of membrane fatty acids, particularly oleic acid, crucial for hyphal morphogenesis [67]. The ions released by the NPs inside the cell can damage lipids, DNA, proteins, and various enzymes, disrupting their structures [68]. Additionally, these ions may inhibit protein synthesis. Jalal et al. demonstrated that Ag NPs significantly reduce the synthesis of hydrolytic enzymes such as phospholipases, proteinases, lipases, and hemolysins in *C. albicans* [62]. Furthermore, ions from the NPs can induce oxidative stress and the production of free radicals like hydrogen peroxide (H_2O_2), superoxide (O^{2-}), and hydroxyl (OH) within the fungal cell [69]. These free radicals can damage the mitochondrial membrane, accelerating cell death. Moreover, metal ions can disrupt the electron transport chain in the membrane [70]. In research by Wani et al., Au NPs were found to inhibit the activity of the H^+_ATPase pump, a crucial protein pump for Candida, thereby affecting the normal membrane structure [71]. Overall, the diverse actions of metal NPs can effectively destroy fungi, including those resistant to drugs (**Figure 2**).

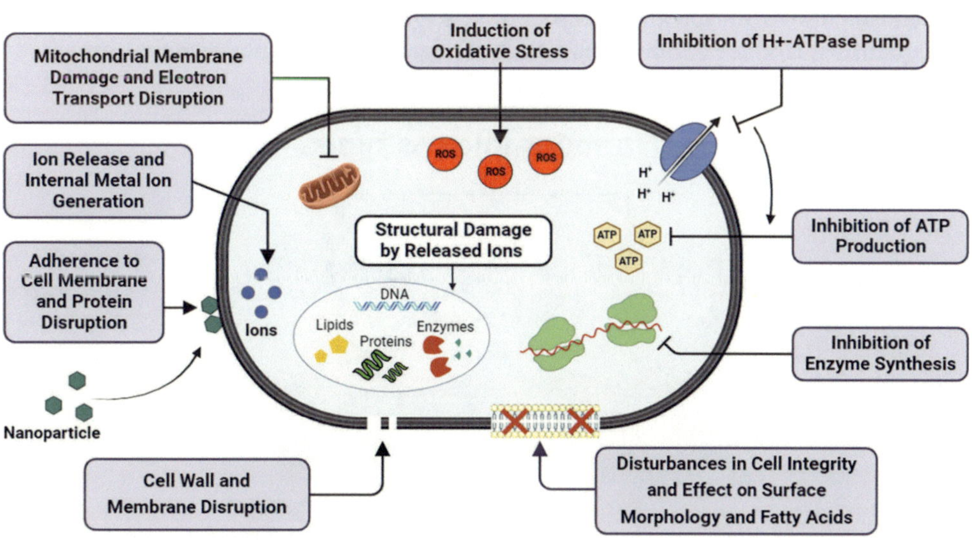

Figure 2.
Mechanism of antifungal activity of metal NPs.

2.1 Metal nanocomplexes

Nanocomplexes present an innovative approach in the realm of nanotechnology, particularly in combating fungal infections such as *C. albicans*. These complexes comprise combinations of multiple NPs, with at least one component being in the nanometer scale [72]. Metal nanocomplexes primarily exist in core-shell or doping states. In the core-shell configuration, one NP constitutes the core of the nanocomplex, around which another NP is layered to form the shell [73]. In the doping mode, one NP acts as the core, and during the doping process, another NP is deposited onto the core at discrete points (**Figure 3**) [74].

It is possible for nanocomplexes to contain more than two types of NPs [75]. In such cases, the resulting nanocomplex exhibits the distinct characteristics of each constituent. Consequently, the properties of the nanocomplex can be tailored and enhanced to meet specific requirements [76]. Various studies have demonstrated that nanocomplexes can significantly eradicate the *C. albicans* fungus more effectively than using their components individually [77]. Owing to the strong antifungal properties of Ag, Au, zinc, and iron NPs, these are frequently utilized in antifungal nanocomplexes. These NPs can either augment their antifungal properties when combined with other NPs or be utilized simultaneously to enhance the overall antifungal activity of the nanocomplex [78, 79].

In a study by Padilla-Cruz et al., a green synthesis method was utilized to fabricate an Ag-iron nanocomplex, which exhibited magnetic properties due to iron. This complex demonstrated greater efficacy in eliminating *C. albicans* than either Ag or iron NPs alone [77]. Similarly, an Ag-nickel nanocomplex exhibited high antifungal activity, even against fluconazole-resistant strains. It inhibited hyphae formation and biofilm development while disrupting membrane function and inducing oxidative stress [12]. Shinde et al. observed that ZnO NPs doped with Ag were more effective than ZnO alone in eradicating *C. albicans* [80].

Studies suggest that nanocomplexes, similar to metal NPs, can eradicate *C. albicans* through multiple mechanisms. These mechanisms employed by nanocomplexes mirror those of individual metal NPs. Initially, nanocomplexes adhere to the fungal cell wall, causing its disruption and subsequent leakage of intracellular substances. They subsequently introduce various ions into the fungal cell [77]. The presence of these

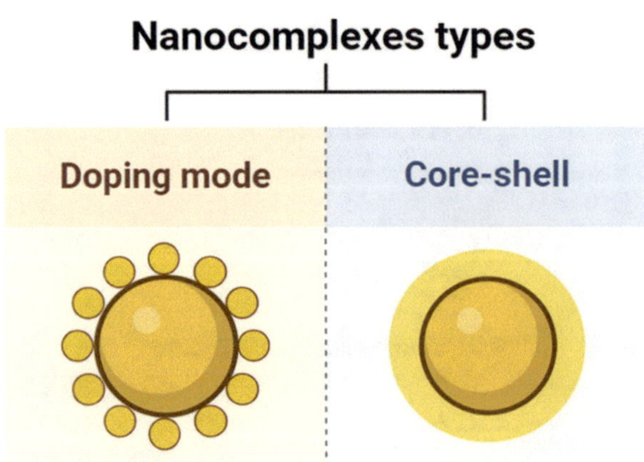

Figure 3.
Nanocomplexes types.

ions damages various cell components, such as proteins and DNA, and induces oxidative stress, further compromising the cell [78]. Consequently, the cumulative damage leads to the destruction of the fungal cell. Due to the presence of multiple types of NPs, nanocomplexes exhibit enhanced effectiveness against *C. albicans* compared to individual NPs. In some cases, the inclusion of specific NPs in the nanocomplex has been observed to mitigate the toxicity of the complex on healthy cells [81].

3. Mesoporous silica NPs

Mesoporous silica NPs (MSNs) are extensively employed in drug delivery systems owing to their distinctive properties. Although they inherently lack antifungal properties, their mesoporous structure make them excellent carriers for various drugs and compounds [82]. Factors such as temperature, concentration, reaction pH, and silica source influence the pore size and overall size of these NPs [83].

MSNs are known for their high chemical and thermal stability, as well as their biocompatibility. They possess a large surface area, and their pore sizes are adjustable, accommodating different drugs [84]. The silanol groups on MSNs can be chemically modified to attach specific drugs to the NPs' surfaces (**Figure 4**) [85].

In the context of *C. albicans*, limited studies have explored the utilization of MSNs. Research by Mas et al. [86] and Montazeri et al. [87] demonstrated that MSNs could enhance the antifungal efficacy of tebuconazole and econazole, respectively. These studies suggest that MSNs can improve drug penetration into fungal cells, thereby boosting antifungal activity against *C. albicans*. Qasim et al. synthesized Ag NPs embedded MSNs, which exhibited anti-Candida activity [88].

Interestingly, MSNs capable of releasing nitric oxide (NO) have been shown to disrupt *C. albicans* biofilms without harming fibroblast cells, attributed to NO release [89]. Kesarwani et al. found that while PEGylated silica NPs alone did not exhibit antifungal activity against *C. albicans*, their conjugation with the antifungal drug caspofungin resulted in effective antifungal action. Additionally, these synthesized NPs were non-toxic to human neutrophil cells [90].

In summary, MSNs are promising carriers for antifungal drugs, enhancing their effectiveness against *C. albicans* while maintaining biocompatibility and minimizing toxicity to human cells.

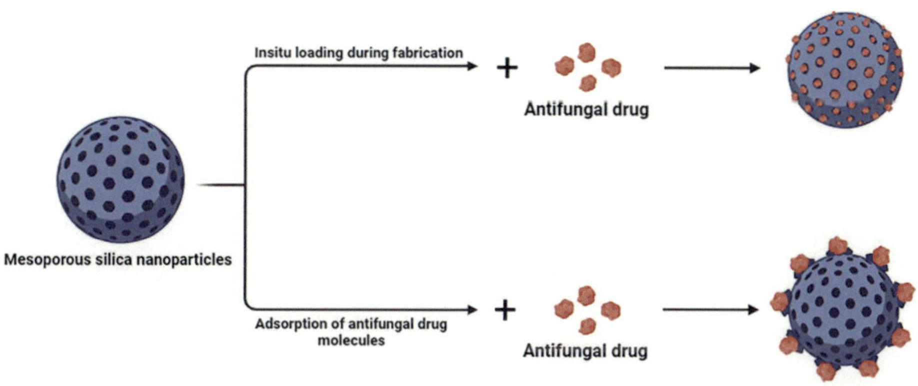

Figure 4.
Mechanisms of drug delivery in MSNs.

4. Liposomal NPs

Liposomes have been employed as carriers for hydrophobic and poorly soluble drugs, showcasing their ability to reduce side effects and mitigate the toxicity of specific medications [91, 92]. The primary constituents of these NPs are phospholipids, arranged in a bilayer structure owing to their amphipathic properties. Upon exposure to water, they form vesicles, enhancing the solubility and stability of anticancer drugs when incorporated into their structure. Notably, liposomes exhibit the capability to encapsulate both hydrophobic and hydrophilic drugs (**Figure 5**) [10]. Additionally, liposomes enable a gradual release of the encapsulated drug, leading to sustained exposure to affected areas and heightened efficacy [93–95].

Liposomal NPs show significant promise in enhancing antifungal activity, improving drug solubility, decreasing toxicity, and potentially mitigating the development of resistance [96]. The utilization of this drug delivery system for microbiological control, particularly as a strategy to inhibit pathogenic microorganisms, is widely acknowledged, especially in combating significant microorganisms that affect humans, such as Candida spp. The scientific literature extensively documents essential research based on the utilization of liposomal formulations for drug delivery in both in vitro and in vivo experimental studies. These efforts aim to control Candida species, contributing to the application of liposomes in candidiasis therapy.

In fact, due to their biocompatibility, biodegradability, non-toxicity, and advantageous physical properties that allow for convenient modifications of surface charge and size, there has been a significant increase in U.S. FDA-approved liposomal or lipid-based nanodrugs since the 1990s. Additionally, numerous others are currently in various stages of preclinical and clinical development. The synthesis and development of new liposomes have been extensively studied in recent years [97].

Gortzi et al. studied the antifungal activities of *Origanum dictamnus* extract with the aim of evaluating the inhibition of *C. albicans*, *Candida krusei*, and *Candida tropicalis* before and after encapsulation in liposomes. The results revealed significant differences in the inhibitory zone diameters when comparing the extract loaded into liposomes with the free extract for all Candida spp. strains. Notably, no inhibitory effects were observed in free liposomes, suggesting that the enhanced activity of the *Origanum dictamnus* extract was attributed to its delivery by the created liposomes [17].

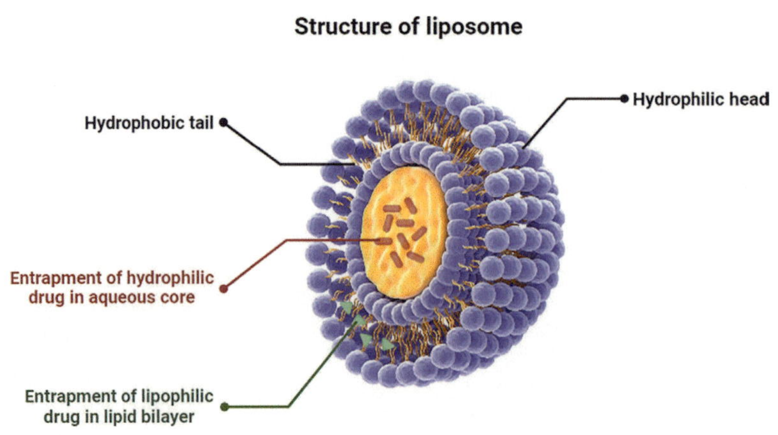

Figure 5.
Structure of liposome.

In 2018, Veloso et al. conducted a study titled "Intravenous delivery of a liposomal formulation of voriconazole improves drug pharmacokinetics, tissue distribution, and enhances antifungal activity". The study concluded that the liposomal formulation significantly promotes the accumulation of voriconazole in the liver and kidneys while safeguarding the drug from biological degradation. Consequently, the liposomal voriconazole for intravenous delivery was suggested as an alternative and effective treatment approach for systemic fungal infections, including those by *C. albicans* [98].

In summary, liposomes exhibit significant therapeutic potential across various domains within health sciences, serving as a pivotal platform for encapsulating drugs with antifungal properties, notably in the context of candidiasis treatment. The provided scientific evidence emphasizes the versatility of this nanostructured drug delivery system. It excels in utilizing materials with low toxicity, ensuring compatibility with living tissues. Additionally, liposomes demonstrate the ability to incorporate drugs with diverse solubility profiles, presenting a strategic approach to candidiasis therapy.

5. Polymeric NPs

Polymeric NPs (PNs), within the spectrum of nanostructured systems, emerge as particularly auspicious nanocarriers currently in development. Characterized by an average diameter falling between 10 and 1000 nm, these biomaterials are widely favored due to their uncomplicated design, compatibility with biological systems, and diverse array of structural characteristics. Polymeric nano-systems can be produced from diverse natural or synthetic starting materials, encompassing collagen, chitosan, gelatin, albumin, as well as polyethylene glycol, polylactic acid, poly(lactic-co-glycolic acid) (PLGA), polylactic acid (PLA), or polycaprolactone (PCL) [11, 99].

Polymer NPs are generally divided into nanocapsules and nanospheres based on their structural form. Nanocapsules comprise a core that dissolves the drug, encapsulated within a polymer shell that regulates its release. On the other hand, nanospheres form a cohesive network of polymers, housing drugs either internally or adhering to the surface (**Figure 6**) [100].

Various polymer options can be selected to generate PNs in order to control the physical and chemical characteristics of the system. These characteristics include solubility, surface load, incorporation efficiency, and release profile, aiming to

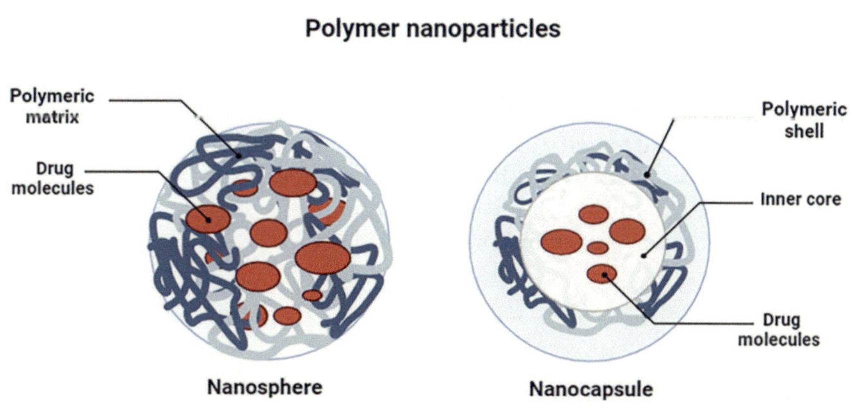

Figure 6.
Types of polymer NPs.

enhance and optimize the performance of these systems within living organisms. The objective of utilizing NP-based treatment for candidiasis is to enhance therapeutic effectiveness and penetration, reduce toxicity, target-specific action, and mitigate drug-related limitations [101].

PNs can be used to improve the efficiency of treatment in opportunistic yeast infections such as *C. albicans* [102]. Given the antimicrobial capabilities of chitosan, a majority of studies have employed this biopolymer in the formulation of nanoscale polymeric systems. Costa et al. created chitosan NPs designed for the simultaneous delivery of miconazole and farnesol to address vulvovaginal candidiasis, primarily caused by the opportunistic fungal strain *C. albicans*. Their findings indicated that the chitosan NPs incorporating both miconazole and farnesol successfully hindered fungal growth. Moreover, chitosan NPs containing farnesol exhibited the ability to reduce the pathogenicity of the infection, as evidenced by the absence of inflammation [103]. Similarly, Charanteja Reddy et al. designed chitosan NPs that encapsulate itraconazole, presenting a potential solution against *C. neoformans*, *C. albicans*, and *Aspergillus fumigatus*. The formulation strategy for itraconazole in these NPs serves to extend the presence of therapeutic drug concentrations in the bloodstream, thereby reducing the frequency of dosage and improving drug efficacy [104]. Panwar et al. formulated chitosan NPs encapsulating farnesol that displayed a favorable positive zeta potential. This characteristic facilitated their binding to the negatively charged membranes of fungi, leading to the disruption of membrane integrity. Consequently, this disruption caused intracellular material leakage and inhibited the formation of biofilms [105]. Also, chitosan has the ability to penetrate the cell wall of fungi and interact with its DNA. This interaction results in the inhibition of mRNA synthesis and the disruption of the production of crucial fungal proteins and enzymes [106]. In another study, Suwan et al. designed silver NPs by green synthesis using aqueous extract of *Psidium gujava* as a reducing agent. Their results showed that coating silver NPs with poloxamer polymer micelles in the right ratio could reduce the size of NPs and significantly prevent the aggregation of silver NPs. The obtained coated silver NPs were effective in inhibiting *C. albicans* [107].

6. Conclusion

The escalating rise in resistant species of *C. albicans* necessitates more effective drugs and treatments to eradicate the disease, and NPs emerge as a viable solution for this purpose. NP can exhibit antifungal activity on their own or synergize with antifungal agents to enhance efficacy and reduce the effective drug dose. Further research is essential to explore NPs that can specifically target *C. albicans*. An important challenge is assessing the toxicity of NPs, a factor that should be carefully considered in the design of antifungal drugs. While the antifungal efficacy of NPs in the in vitro environment is well-established, additional studies in the in vivo setting are imperative to comprehend their impact and potential side effects in vivo.

Conflict of interest

The authors declare no conflict of interest.

Author details

Sobhan Mortazavi-Derazkola[1*], Seyedeh Masoumeh Ghoreishi[2], Pouria Mohammadparast-Tabas[3,4], Hamed Aramjoo[3] and Azar Bazrgaran[5]

1 Medical Toxicology and Drug Abuse Research Center (MTDRC), Birjand University of Medical Sciences, Birjand, Iran

2 Cellular and Molecular Biology Research Center, Health Research Institute, Babol University of Medical Sciences, Babol, Iran

3 Faculty of Medicine, Department of Medical Biotechnology, Birjand University of Medical Science, Birjand, Iran

4 Student Research Committee, Birjand University of Medical Sciences, Birjand, Iran

5 Department of Medical Microbiology, School of Medicine, Shahid Beheshti University of Medical Sciences, Tehran, Iran

*Address all correspondence to: s.mortazavi23@yahoo.com

References

[1] Castillo HAP, Castellanos LNM, Chamorro RM, Martínez RR, Borunda EO. Nanoparticles as new therapeutic agents against *Candida albicans*. In: *Candida albicans*. London, UK: IntechOpen; 2018

[2] Raja NS. Epidemiology, risk factors, treatment and outcome of Candida bloodstream infections because of *Candida albicans* and Candida non-albicans in two district general hospitals in the United Kingdom. International Journal of Clinical Practice. 2021;**75**(1):e13655

[3] Ayaal F, Chehri K. Antifungal activity of Au, Ag, Tio_2, Ch, Pd, Se, and Zno nanoparticles against *Candida albicans*: A review. Plant Archives. 2019;**19**(1):33-44

[4] Carmo PHF, Garcia MT, Figueiredo-Godoi LMA, Lage ACP, Silva NS, Junqueira JC. Metal nanoparticles to combat *Candida albicans* infections: An update. Microorganisms. 2023;**11**(1):138

[5] Moran GP, Coleman DC, Sullivan DJ. *Candida albicans* versus *Candida dubliniensis*: Why is *C. albicans* more pathogenic? International Journal of Microbiology. 2012;**2012**:205921

[6] Dadar M, Tiwari R, Karthik K, Chakraborty S, Shahali Y, Dhama K. *Candida albicans*-biology, molecular characterization, pathogenicity, and advances in diagnosis and control–an update. Microbial Pathogenesis. 2018;**117**:128-138

[7] Joshi KM, Shelar A, Kasabe U, Nikam LK, Pawar RA, Sangshetti J, et al. Biofilm inhibition in *Candida albicans* with biogenic hierarchical zinc-oxide nanoparticles. Biomaterials Advances. 2022;**134**:112592

[8] Kim K-J, Sung WS, Suh BK, Moon S-K, Choi J-S, Kim JG, et al. Antifungal activity and mode of action of silver nano-particles on *Candida albicans*. Biometals. 2009;**22**:235-242

[9] Mba IE, Nweze EI. The use of nanoparticles as alternative therapeutic agents against Candida infections: An up-to-date overview and future perspectives. World Journal of Microbiology and Biotechnology. 2020;**36**:1-20

[10] Yingchoncharoen P, Kalinowski DS, Richardson DR. Lipid-based drug delivery systems in cancer therapy: What is available and what is yet to come. Pharmacological Reviews. 2016;**68**(3):701-787

[11] Bitencourt PE, Ferreira LM, Cargnelutti LO, Denardi L, Boligon A, Fleck M, et al. A new biodegradable polymeric nanoparticle formulation containing *Syzygium cumini*: Phytochemical profile, antioxidant and antifungal activity and *in vivo* toxicity. Industrial Crops and Products. 2016;**83**:400-407

[12] Kamli MR, Alzahrani EA, Albukhari SM, Ahmad A, Sabir JS, Malik MA. Combination effect of novel bimetallic Ag-Ni nanoparticles with fluconazole against *Candida albicans*. Journal of Fungi. 2022;**8**(7):733

[13] Abdallah BM, Ali EM. Green synthesis of silver nanoparticles using the lotus lalambensis aqueous leaf extract and their anti-candidal activity against oral candidiasis. ACS Omega. 2021;**6**(12):8151-8162

[14] Zhang H, Zhang Y, Li Y, Hu M, Rong Z, Meng L, et al. A novel silver

nanoparticles-decorated metal-organic framework with rapid and sustained antimicrobial activity against drug-resistant *Candida albicans* through synergistic Chemodynamic and Sonodynamic therapy. Advanced Therapeutics. 2023;**6**(8):2300074

[15] Roque-Borda CA, Da Silva PB, Rodrigues MC, Di Filippo LD, Duarte JL, Chorilli M, et al. Pharmaceutical nanotechnology: Antimicrobial peptides as potential new drugs against WHO list of critical, high, and medium priority bacteria. European Journal of Medicinal Chemistry. 2022;**241**:114640

[16] Ahmad A, Wei Y, Syed F, Tahir K, Taj R, Khan AU, et al. Amphotericin B-conjugated biogenic silver nanoparticles as an innovative strategy for fungal infections. Microbial Pathogenesis. 2016;**99**:271-281

[17] Gortzi O, Lalas S, Chinou I, Tsaknis J. Evaluation of the antimicrobial and antioxidant activities of *Origanum dictamnus* extracts before and after encapsulation in liposomes. Molecules. 2007;**12**(5):932-945

[18] Balabathula P, Whaley SG, Janagam DR, Mittal NK, Mandal B, Thoma LA, et al. Lyophilized iron oxide nanoparticles encapsulated in amphotericin B: A novel targeted nano drug delivery system for the treatment of systemic fungal infections. Pharmaceutics. 2020;**12**(3):247

[19] Liu S, Xu X, Ye J, Wang J, Wang Q, Liu Z, et al. Metal-coordinated nanodrugs based on natural products for cancer theranostics. Chemical Engineering Journal. 2023;**456**:140892

[20] Amiri MR, Alavi M, Taran M, Kahrizi D. Antibacterial, antifungal, antiviral, and photocatalytic activities of TiO_2 nanoparticles, nanocomposites, and bio-nanocomposites: Recent advances and challenges. Journal of Public Health Research. 2022;**11**(2):22799036221104151

[21] Mohamed AA, Abu-Elghait M, Ahmed NE, Salem SS. Eco-friendly mycogenic synthesis of ZnO and CuO nanoparticles for *in vitro* antibacterial, antibiofilm, and antifungal applications. Biological Trace Element Research. 2021;**199**:2788-2799

[22] Jamkhande PG, Ghule NW, Bamer AH, Kalaskar MG. Metal nanoparticles synthesis: An overview on methods of preparation, advantages and disadvantages, and applications. Journal of Drug Delivery Science and Technology. 2019;**53**:101174

[23] Shnoudeh AJ, Hamad I, Abdo RW, Qadumii L, Jaber AY, Surchi HS, et al. Synthesis, characterization, and applications of metal nanoparticles. In: Biomaterials and Bionanotechnology. Netherland: Elsevier; 2019. pp. 527-612

[24] Ijaz I, Gilani E, Nazir A, Bukhari A. Detail review on chemical, physical and green synthesis, classification, characterizations and applications of nanoparticles. Green Chemistry Letters and Reviews. 2020;**13**(3):223-245

[25] Zhang D, Ma X-l, Gu Y, Huang H, Zhang G-w. Green synthesis of metallic nanoparticles and their potential applications to treat cancer. Frontiers in Chemistry. 2020;**8**:799

[26] Pathania D, Sharma M, Thakur P, Chaudhary V, Kaushik A, Furukawa H, et al. Exploring phytochemical composition, photocatalytic, antibacterial, and antifungal efficacies of Au NPs supported by *Cymbopogon flexuosus* essential oil. Scientific Reports. 2022;**12**(1):14249

[27] Aflakian F, Mirzavi F, Aiyelabegan HT, Soleimani A, Navashenaq JG, Karimi-Sani I, et al. Nanoparticles-based therapeutics for the management of bacterial infections: A special emphasis on FDA approved products and clinical trials. European Journal of Pharmaceutical Sciences. 2023;**188**:106515

[28] Graczyk A, Pawlowska R, Jedrzejczyk D, Chworos A. Gold nanoparticles in conjunction with nucleic acids as a modern molecular system for cellular delivery. Molecules. 2020;**25**(1):204

[29] Vigderman L, Zubarev ER. Therapeutic platforms based on gold nanoparticles and their covalent conjugates with drug molecules. Advanced Drug Delivery Reviews. 2013;**65**(5):663-676

[30] Osonga FJ, Akgul A, Yazgan I, Akgul A, Eshun GB, Sakhaee L, et al. Size and shape-dependent antimicrobial activities of silver and gold nanoparticles: A model study as potential fungicides. Molecules. 2020;**25**(11):2682

[31] Haji Esmaeil Hajjar F, Jebali A, Hekmatimoghaddam S. The inhibition of *Candida albicans* secreted aspartyl proteinase by triangular gold nanoparticles. Nanomedicine Journal. 2015;**2**(1):54-59

[32] Rahimi H, Roudbarmohammadi S, Delavari HH, Roudbary M. Antifungal effects of indolicidin-conjugated gold nanoparticles against fluconazole-resistant strains of *Candida albicans* isolated from patients with burn infection. International Journal of Nanomedicine. 2019;**14**:5323-5338

[33] Salehi Z, Fattahi A, Lotfali E, Kazemi A, Shakeri-Zadeh A, Nasrollahi SA. Susceptibility pattern of caspofungin-coated gold nanoparticles against clinically important Candida species. Advanced Pharmaceutical Bulletin. 2021;**11**(4):693

[34] Kareem HA, Samaka HM. Evaluation of the effect of the gold nanoparticles prepared by green chemistry on the treatment of cutaneous candidiasis. Current Medical Mycology. 2021;**7**(1):1

[35] Azizi-Lalabadi M, Garavand F, Jafari SM. Incorporation of silver nanoparticles into active antimicrobial nanocomposites: Release behavior, analyzing techniques, applications and safety issues. Advances in Colloid and Interface Science. 2021;**293**:102440

[36] Gul AR, Shaheen F, Rafique R, Bal J, Waseem S, Park TJ. Grass-mediated biogenic synthesis of silver nanoparticles and their drug delivery evaluation: A biocompatible anti-cancer therapy. Chemical Engineering Journal. 2021;**407**:127202

[37] Tanwar J, Sharma M, Parmar A, Tehri N, Verma N, Gahlaut A, et al. Antibacterial potential of silver nanoparticles against multidrug resistant bacterial isolates from blood cultures. Inorganic and Nano-Metal Chemistry. 2020;**50**(11):1150-1156

[38] Téllez-de-Jesús DG, Flores-Lopez N, Cervantes-Chávez J, Hernández-Martínez A. Antibacterial and antifungal activities of encapsulated Au and Ag nanoparticles synthesized using *Argemone mexicana* L extract, against antibiotic-resistant bacteria and *Candida albicans*. Surfaces and Interfaces. 2021;**27**:101456

[39] Alimehr S, Abad HSE, Shahverdi A, Hashemi J, Zomorodian K, Moazeni M, et al. Comparison of difference between fluconazole and silver nanoparticles in antimicrobial effect on fluconazole-resistant *Candida albicans* strains.

Archives of Pediatric Infectious Diseases. 2015;**3**(2):e21481

[40] Jia D, Sun W. Silver nanoparticles offer a synergistic effect with fluconazole against fluconazole-resistant *Candida albicans* by abrogating drug efflux pumps and increasing endogenous ROS. Infection, Genetics and Evolution. 2021;**93**:104937

[41] Mohammadi M, Shahisaraee SA, Tavajjohi A, Pournoori N, Muhammadnejad S, Mohammadi SR, et al. Green synthesis of silver nanoparticles using Zingiber officinale and Thymus vulgaris extracts: Characterisation, cell cytotoxicity, and its antifungal activity against *Candida albicans* in comparison to fluconazole. IET Nanobiotechnology. 2019;**13**(2):114-119

[42] Nasiri S, Nasiri S. Biosynthesis of silver nanoparticles using Carum carvi extract and its inhibitory effect on growth of *Candida albicans*. Avicenna Journal of Medical Biochemistry. 2016;**4**(2):8-37504

[43] Öztürk BY, Gürsu BY, Dağ İ. Antibiofilm and antimicrobial activities of green synthesized silver nanoparticles using marine red algae *Gelidium corneum*. Process Biochemistry. 2020;**89**:208-219

[44] Jin S-E, Jin H-E. Antimicrobial activity of zinc oxide nano/microparticles and their combinations against pathogenic microorganisms for biomedical applications: From physicochemical characteristics to pharmacological aspects. Nanomaterials. 2021;**11**(2):263

[45] Hajar AA, Dakhili M, Saghazadeh M, Aghaei S, Nazari R. Synergistic antifungal effect of fluconazole combined with ZnO nanoparticles against *Candida albicans* strains from vaginal candidiasis. Medical Laboratory Journal. 2020;**14**(3):26-32

[46] Hosseini SS, Joshaghani H, Shokohi T, Ahmadi A, Mehrbakhsh Z. Antifungal activity of ZnO nanoparticles and nystatin and downregulation of SAP1-3 genes expression in fluconazole-resistant *Candida albicans* isolates from vulvovaginal candidiasis. Infection and Drug Resistance. 2020;**13**:385-394

[47] Nasiri S, Mahmoudvand H, Shakibaei M, Mousavi SAH, Sepahvand A. Antifungal effects of zinc nanoparticles green synthesized by Lavandula angustifolia extract, alone and combined with nystatin against *Candida albicans*, a major cause of oral candidiasis. Journal of Herbmed Pharmacology. 2022;**11**(4):540-545

[48] Pillai AM, Sivasankarapillai VS, Rahdar A, Joseph J, Sadeghfar F, Rajesh K, et al. Green synthesis and characterization of zinc oxide nanoparticles with antibacterial and antifungal activity. Journal of Molecular Structure. 2020;**1211**:128107

[49] Low LE, Lim HP, Ong YS, Siva SP, Sia CS, Goh B-H, et al. Stimuli-controllable iron oxide nanoparticle assemblies: Design, manipulation and bio-applications. Journal of Controlled Release. 2022;**345**:231-274

[50] Al-Husseini A, Sih B, Al-Araji A. Effect of iron oxide nanoparticles (Fe_2O_3) on *Candida albicans* and Candida Glabrata. NVEO-Natural Volatiles & Essential Oils Journal. 2021;**8**:12394-12405

[51] Alangari A, Alqahtani MS, Mateen A, Kalam MA, Alshememry A, Ali R, et al. Iron oxide nanoparticles: Preparation, characterization, and assessment of antimicrobial and anticancer activity.

Adsorption Science & Technology. 2022;**2022**:1-9

[52] Sidkey N. Biosynthesis, characterization and antimicrobial activity of iron oxide nanoparticles synthesized by fungi. Al-Azhar Journal of Pharmaceutical Sciences. 2020;**62**(2):164-179

[53] Elemike EE, Nna PJ, Ikenweke C, Onwudiwe D, Omotade ET, Singh M. Synthesis, characterization, anti-cancer and antimicrobial studies of iron oxide nanoparticles mediated by *Terminalia catappa* (Indian almond) leaf extract. Inorganic Chemistry Communications. 2023;**155**:111048

[54] Farouk F, Abdelmageed M, Azam Ansari M, Azzazy HM. Synthesis of magnetic iron oxide nanoparticles using pulp and seed aqueous extract of Citrullus colocynth and evaluation of their antimicrobial activity. Biotechnology Letters. 2020;**42**:231-240

[55] Guisbiers G, Lara HH, Mendoza-Cruz R, Naranjo G, Vincent BA, Peralta XG, et al. Inhibition of *Candida albicans* biofilm by pure selenium nanoparticles synthesized by pulsed laser ablation in liquids. Nanomedicine: Nanotechnology, Biology and Medicine. 2017;**13**(3):1095-1103

[56] Moradpoor H, Safaei M, Golshah A, Mozaffari HR, Sharifi R, Imani MM, et al. Green synthesis and antifungal effect of titanium dioxide nanoparticles on oral *Candida albicans* pathogen. Inorganic Chemistry Communications. 2021;**130**:108748

[57] Jeba R, Radhika S, Padma CM, Ascar Davix X. Structural, optical, thermal, magnetic properties of zirconia nano-rods and their photocatalytic and antimicrobial properties. Journal of Water and Environmental Nanotechnology. 2021;**6**(3):252-264

[58] Imani MM, Safaei M, Moradpoor H, Rezaei R, Golshah A, Rezaei F, et al. Optimum synthesis of CuO nanoparticles with the highest antifungal activity against oral pathogen *Candida albicans*. Journal of Applied Pharmaceutical Science. 2020;**10**(2):021-025

[59] Kong F, Wang J, Han R, Ji S, Yue J, Wang Y, et al. Antifungal activity of magnesium oxide nanoparticles: Effect on the growth and key virulence factors of *Candida albicans*. Mycopathologia. 2020;**185**:485-494

[60] Halbandge SD, Jadhav AK, Jangid PM, Shelar AV, Patil RH, Karuppayil SM. Molecular targets of biofabricated silver nanoparticles in *Candida albicans*. The Journal of Antibiotics. 2019;**72**(8):640-644

[61] Muthamil S, Devi VA, Balasubramaniam B, Balamurugan K, Pandian SK. Green synthesized silver nanoparticles demonstrating enhanced *in vitro* and *in vivo* antibiofilm activity against Candida spp. Journal of Basic Microbiology. 2018;**58**(4):343-357

[62] Jalal M, Ansari MA, Alzohairy MA, Ali SG, Khan HM, Almatroudi A, et al. Anticandidal activity of biosynthesized silver nanoparticles: Effect on growth, cell morphology, and key virulence attributes of Candida species. International Journal of Nanomedicine. 2019;**14**:4667-4679

[63] Arya G, Kumari RM, Pundir R, Chatterjee S, Gupta N, Kumar A, et al. Versatile biomedical potential of biosynthesized silver nanoparticles from Acacia nilotica bark. Journal of Applied Biomedicine. 2019;**17**(2):115-124

[64] Gutiérrez JA, Caballero S, Díaz LA, Guerrero MA, Ruiz J, Ortiz CC. High antifungal activity against candida species of monometallic and bimetallic

nanoparticles synthesized in nanoreactors. ACS Biomaterials Science & Engineering. 2018;**4**(2):647-653

[65] Al-Sahli SA, Al-Otibi F, Alharbi RI, Amina M, Al Musayeib NM. Silver nanoparticles improve the fungicidal properties of Rhazya stricta decne aqueous extract against plant pathogens. Scientific Reports. 2024;**14**(1):1297

[66] Lara HH, Romero-Urbina DG, Pierce C, Lopez-Ribot JL, Arellano-Jiménez MJ, Jose-Yacaman M. Effect of silver nanoparticles on *Candida albicans* biofilms: An ultrastructural study. Journal of Nanobiotechnology. 2015;**13**(1):1-12

[67] Radhakrishnan VS, Reddy Mudiam MK, Kumar M, Dwivedi SP, Singh SP, Prasad T. Silver nanoparticles induced alterations in multiple cellular targets, which are critical for drug susceptibilities and pathogenicity in fungal pathogen (*Candida albicans*). International Journal of Nanomedicine. 2018;**13**:2647-2663

[68] Guilger-Casagrande M, Germano-Costa T, Pasquoto-Stigliani T, Fraceto LF, Lima R. Biosynthesis of silver nanoparticles employing *Trichoderma harzianum* with enzymatic stimulation for the control of *Sclerotinia sclerotiorum*. Scientific Reports. 2019;**9**(1):14351

[69] Is H, Lee J, Hwang JH, Kim KJ, Lee DG. Silver nanoparticles induce apoptotic cell death in *Candida albicans* through the increase of hydroxyl radicals. The FEBS Journal. 2012;**279**(7):1327-1338

[70] Umamaheswari K, Abirami M. Assessment of antifungal action mechanism of green synthesized gold nanoparticles (AuNPs) using *Allium sativum* on Candida species. Materials Letters. 2023;**333**:133616

[71] Wani IA, Ahmad T. Size and shape dependant antifungal activity of gold nanoparticles: A case study of Candida. Colloids and surfaces B: Biointerfaces. 2013;**101**:162-170

[72] Yamashita M. Next generation multifunctional nano-science of advanced metal complexes with quantum effect and nonlinearity. Bulletin of the Chemical Society of Japan. 2021;**94**(1):209-264

[73] Wei B, Zhou J, Yao Z, Haidry AA, Qian K, Lin H, et al. Excellent microwave absorption property of nano-Ni coated hollow silicon carbide core-shell spheres. Applied Surface Science. 2020;**508**:145261

[74] Saxena V, Pandey LM. Bimetallic assembly of Fe (III) doped ZnO as an effective nanoantibiotic and its ROS independent antibacterial mechanism. Journal of Trace Elements in Medicine and Biology. 2020;**57**:126416

[75] Ye Z, Padilla JA, Xuriguera E, Brillas E, Sirés I. Magnetic MIL (Fe)-type MOF-derived N-doped nano-ZVI@C rods as heterogeneous catalyst for the electro-Fenton degradation of gemfibrozil in a complex aqueous matrix. Applied Catalysis B: Environmental. 2020;**266**:118604

[76] Rezaei M, Nezamzadeh-Ejhieha A. The ZnO-NiO nano-composite: A brief characterization, kinetic and thermodynamic study and study the Arrhenius model on the sulfasalazine photodegradation. International Journal of Hydrogen Energy. 2020;**45**(46):24749-24764

[77] Padilla-Cruz A, Garza-Cervantes J, Vasto-Anzaldo XG, García-Rivas G, León-Buitimea A, Morones-Ramírez J. Synthesis and design of Ag–Fe bimetallic nanoparticles as antimicrobial synergistic

combination therapies against clinically relevant pathogens. Scientific Reports. 2021;**11**(1):5351

[78] Noohpisheh Z, Amiri H, Farhadi S, Mohammadi-Gholami A. Green synthesis of Ag-ZnO nanocomposites using *Trigonella foenum*-graecum leaf extract and their antibacterial, antifungal, antioxidant and photocatalytic properties. Spectrochimica Acta Part A: Molecular and Biomolecular Spectroscopy. 2020;**240**:118595

[79] Parthiban E, Kalaivasan N, Sudarsan S. A study of magnetic, antibacterial and antifungal behaviour of a novel gold anchor of polyaniline/itaconic acid/Fe_3O_4 hybrid nanocomposite: Synthesis and characterization. Arabian Journal of Chemistry. 2020;**13**(3):4751-4763

[80] Shinde RS, More RA, Adole VA, Koli PB, Pawar TB, Jagdale BS, et al. Design, fabrication, antitubercular, antibacterial, antifungal and antioxidant study of silver doped ZnO and CuO nano candidates: A comparative pharmacological study. Current Research in Green and Sustainable Chemistry. 2021;**4**:100138

[81] Sayed MA, El-Rahman TMA, Abdelsalam H, Ali AM, Hamdy MM, Badr YA, et al. Attractive study of the antimicrobial, antiviral, and cytotoxic activity of novel synthesized silver chromite nanocomposites. BMC Chemistry. 2022;**16**(1):39

[82] Manzano M, Vallet-Regí M. Mesoporous silica nanoparticles for drug delivery. Advanced Functional Materials. 2020;**30**(2):1902634

[83] Vallet-Regí M, Schüth F, Lozano D, Colilla M, Manzano M. Engineering mesoporous silica nanoparticles for drug delivery: Where are we after two decades? Chemical Society Reviews. 2022;**51**(13):5365-5451

[84] Ahmed H, Gomte SS, Prathyusha E, Prabakaran A, Agrawal M, Alexander A. Biomedical applications of mesoporous silica nanoparticles as a drug delivery carrier. Journal of Drug Delivery Science and Technology. 2022;**76**:103729

[85] Mohamed Isa ED, Ahmad H, Abdul Rahman MB, Gill MR. Progress in mesoporous silica nanoparticles as drug delivery agents for cancer treatment. Pharmaceutics. 2021;**13**(2):152

[86] Mas N, Galiana I, Hurtado S, Mondragón L, Bernardos A, Sancenón F, et al. Enhanced antifungal efficacy of tebuconazole using gated pH-driven mesoporous nanoparticles. International Journal of Nanomedicine. 2014;**9**:2597-2606

[87] Montazeri M, Razzaghi-Abyaneh M, Nasrollahi S, Maibach H, Nafisi S. Enhanced topical econazole antifungal efficacy by amine-functionalized silica nanoparticles. Bulletin of Materials Science. 2020;**43**(1):13

[88] Qasim M, Singh BR, Naqvi A, Paik P, Das D. Silver nanoparticles embedded mesoporous SiO2 nanosphere: An effective anticandidal agent against *Candida albicans* 077. Nanotechnology. 2015;**26**(28):285102

[89] Hetrick EM, Shin JH, Paul HS, Schoenfisch MH. Anti-biofilm efficacy of nitric oxide-releasing silica nanoparticles. Biomaterials. 2009;**30**(14):2782-2789

[90] Kesarwani V, Kelly HG, Shankar M, Robinson KJ, Kent SJ, Traven A, et al. Characterization of key bio–nano interactions between organosilica nanoparticles and *Candida albicans*.

ACS Applied Materials & Interfaces. 2019;**11**(38):34676-34687

[91] Allen TM, Cullis PR. Drug delivery systems: Entering the mainstream. Science. 2004;**303**(5665):1818-1822

[92] Chen C, Han D, Cai C, Tang X. An overview of liposome lyophilization and its future potential. Journal of Controlled Release. 2010;**142**(3):299-311

[93] Balasubramanian SV, Straubinger RM. Taxol-lipid interactions: Taxol-dependent effects on the physical properties of model membranes. Biochemistry. 1994;**33**(30):8941-8947

[94] Sharma A, Sharma US. Liposomes in drug delivery: Progress and limitations. International Journal of Pharmaceutics. 1997;**154**(2):123-140

[95] Zhang JA, Xuan T, Parmar M, Ma L, Ugwu S, Ali S, et al. Development and characterization of a novel liposome-based formulation of SN-38. International Journal of Pharmaceutics. 2004;**270**(1-2):93-107

[96] Vera-González N, Bailey-Hytholt CM, Langlois L, de Camargo RF, de Souza Santos EL, Junqueira JC, et al. Anidulafungin liposome nanoparticles exhibit antifungal activity against planktonic and biofilm *Candida albicans*. Journal of Biomedical Materials Research Part A. 2020;**108**(11):2263-2276

[97] Jiang Y, Li W, Wang Z, Lu J. Lipid-based nanotechnology: Liposome. Pharmaceutics. 2023;**16**(1):34

[98] Veloso DF, Benedetti NI, Ávila RI, Bastos TS, Silva TC, Silva MR, et al. Intravenous delivery of a liposomal formulation of voriconazole improves drug pharmacokinetics, tissue distribution, and enhances antifungal activity. Drug Delivery. 2018;**25**(1):1585-1594

[99] Spirescu VA, Chircov C, Grumezescu AM, Andronescu E. Polymeric nanoparticles for antimicrobial therapies: An up-to-date overview. Polymers. 2021;**13**(5):724

[100] Li B, Pan L, Zhang H, Xie L, Wang X, Shou J, et al. Recent developments on using nanomaterials to combat *Candida albicans*. Frontiers in Chemistry. 2021;**9**:813973

[101] Qais FA, Khan MS, Ahmad I, Althubiani AS. Potential of nanoparticles in combating Candida infections. Letters in Drug Design & Discovery. 2019;**16**(5):478-491

[102] Roque L, Castro P, Molpeceres J, Viana AS, Roberto A, Reis C, et al. Bioadhesive polymeric nanoparticles as strategy to improve the treatment of yeast infections in oral cavity: *in-vitro* and *ex-vivo* studies. European Polymer Journal. 2018;**104**:19-31

[103] Fernandes Costa A, Evangelista Araujo D, Santos Cabral M, Teles Brito I, de Menezes B, Leite L, et al. Development, characterization, and *in vitro–in vivo* evaluation of polymeric nanoparticles containing miconazole and farnesol for treatment of vulvovaginal candidiasis. Medical Mycology. 2019;**57**(1):52-62

[104] Reddy Y, Jeganath S, Munikumar U. Formulation and evaluation of chitosan nanoparticles for improved efficacy of itraconazole antifungal drug. Asian Journal of Pharmaceutical and Clinical Research. 2018;**11**:147-152

[105] Panwar R, Pemmaraju SC, Sharma AK, Pruthi V. Efficacy of ferulic acid encapsulated chitosan nanoparticles against *Candida albicans* biofilm. Microbial Pathogenesis. 2016;**95**:21-31

[106] Kong M, Chen XG, Xing K, Park HJ. Antimicrobial properties of chitosan

and mode of action: A state of the art review. International Journal of Food Microbiology. 2010;**144**(1):51-63

[107] Suwan T, Khongkhunthian S, Okonogi S. Antifungal activity of polymeric micelles of silver nanoparticles prepared from *Psidium guajava* aqueous extract. Drug Discoveries & Therapeutics. 2019;**13**(2):62-69